CW00430193

Indirect Restorations

Quintessentials of Dental Practice – 25
Operative Dentistry – 3

Indirect restorations

By
David Bartlett
David Ricketts

Editor-in-Chief: Nairn H F Wilson
Editor Operative Dentistry: Paul A Brunton

Quintessence Publishing Co. Ltd.

London, Berlin, Chicago, Paris, Milan, Barcelona, Istanbul,
São Paulo, Tokyo, New Delhi, Moscow, Prague, Warsaw

British Library Cataloguing in Publication Data

Bartlett, David
 Indirect restorations. - (Quintessentials of dental practice; v. 25)
 1. Crowns (Dentistry)
 I. Title II. Ricketts, David III. Wilson, Nairn H.F.
 617.6'922

ISBN-13: 9781850970781

ISBN-13: 978-1-85097-078-1

Foreword

The successful provision of indirect restrictions is demanding. A diversity of skills, knowledge and experience are required to consistently succeed in this important aspect of clinical practice. Mediocrity in indirect restorations is tantamount to inviting early failure, with the risk of substantial damage to the remaining tooth tissues and the dentition.

Interestingly, failure is the starting point of this latest addition to the *Quintessentials* series – most indirect restorations replacing failed restorations. Against this backdrop, the authors take the reader through the indications and the many, varied intricacies integral to the provision of successful indirect restorations. The text, as has come to be expected of new volumes in the popular *Quintessentials* series, is generously illustrated and peppered with invaluable tips and guidance, tempered by the authors' special interests and expertise in the field.

As indicated by the authors in their Preface, this book is not intended to be a comprehensive tome; it is a succinct text highlighting key considerations, knowledge and understanding for the busy practitioner, let alone the student wishing to avoid information overload. Once read, this book should not be put aside, but placed together with other *Quintessentials* volumes and similar books for ready reference and guidance.

Hopefully, this book will give clinicians new insight and pointers to enhanced success, if not excellence in indirect restorations. This is a handsome, easy-to-read book, promoting a modern evidence-based approach to indirect restorations.

Congratulations to the authors for a job well done.

Nairn Wilson
Editor-in-Chief

Preface

This book is written to guide practitioners and students in the restoration of teeth by means of indirect restorations. Many well written textbooks on this subject already exist. This volume is not intended to be a definitive work; by contrast, it is an overview of key points and issues critical to success with indirect restorations. We have not included conventional and minimal preparation bridgework as there are other books in the *Quintessentials* series covering these topics. But many of the principles in this book can be applied to these areas.

On reading this book the reader will be able to:

- Plan indirect restorations taking into consideration the importance of previous caries experience. The reasons for placing indirect restorations will be reappraised.
- Consider and review the indications for indirect full and partial coverage crowns.
- Appreciate how to place reliable and retentive cores.
- Consider what factors are important when choosing the type of crown and how to select the best materials to use.

The book also:

- Describes the common tooth preparations for crowns and assesses how to achieve the best result.
- Describes how to take a shade, make provisional restorations, record impressions and explains the value of taking interocclusal records.
- Considers aspects of occlusion and explains the relevance of occlusal consideration in the provision of indirect restorations.
- Reviews the problems associated with short clinical crowns and how to manage them.
- Describes when and how to use an articulator.

David Bartlett and David Ricketts
London and Dundee

Acknowledgements

David Ricketts would like to express his gratitude to Catherine Burnett for her assistance with the photography in this book.

Both authors would also like to acknowledge the laboratory technicians who made the crowns illustrated in this book.

Chapter 1
Introduction

Aim

To familiarise the reader with planning indirect restorations, taking into consideration the importance of previous dental history. The reasons for placing indirect restorations are reappraised.

Outcome

On reading this chapter the reader will better understand the importance of prevention and maintaining pulp and periodontal health in the provision of successful indirect restorations.

Introduction

To the reader, it may seem strange that a text on successful indirect restorations should begin with a chapter discussing failures. But in terms of success, it is probably the most important subject as many indirect restorations are replacement restorations. The restorative cycle, once established, will continue unless lessons are learnt from failure events. This chapter will consider the:
- failure of direct and indirect restorations
- maintenance of pulp health
- importance of periodontal health
- importance of pulp vitality.

Why Indirect Restorations?

Most indirect restorations are placed to restore the contour, function and appearance of teeth previously restored with plastic restorations. In restoring broken down or damaged teeth with plastic restorations, it is sometimes difficult to achieve appropriate contact areas (Fig 1-1) and occlusal form (Fig 1-2). Indirect restorations such as crowns, onlays and inlays enable the contact areas and the occlusal form to be controlled in the laboratory. The majority of extensive restorations are placed because of primary caries, or caries adjacent to existing restorations. Others will be placed following a fracture of tooth tissue, classically a cusp fracture associated with an occlusoproximal restoration (Fig 1-3). Relatively few extensive restorations are placed as a consequence of trauma.

Why do Indirect Restorations Fail?

Studies on the failure of indirect restorations indicate that the commonest cause of failure is secondary caries as diagnosed clinically. Other causes

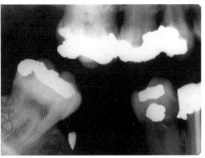

Fig 1-1 Bitewing radiograph showing a ledge on the amalgam restoration in the LR4. This occurred as the LR4 has an extensive defect, making it difficult to develop a tight contact area while keeping the matrix band adapted cervically.

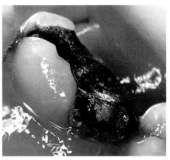

Fig 1-2 Given the extent of this cavity, it is difficult to place an amalgam restoration with adequate occlusal contour.

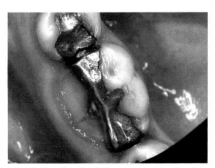

Fig 1-3 The MOD restoration in this lower molar tooth, although not large, has weakened the tooth and the lingual cusp has fractured.

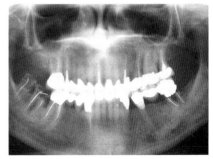

Fig 1-4 Dental panoramic tomogram of a patient with an extensively restored dentition; including multiple indirect restorations. Failure of many of the restorations has been caused by caries, some have been lost (LR7 and 8), and some have been repaired (LL5).

include various forms of mechanical breakdown and failure, together with unacceptable appearance and endodontic and periodontic complications.

Dental Caries

Caries remains the most important disease that affects teeth. It is responsible for most directly placed restorations and their subsequent replacements. Ultimately, when direct restorations are contraindicated, indirect restorations are required, but typically these will not be permanent and will fail because of caries. This is ironic given that dental caries is a preventable disease.

Failures such as those illustrated in Fig 1-4 are preventable. It is important that we learn from such failures, by ensuring that operative dentistry is preventively driven.

Before placing indirect restorations, it is important that the patient's caries risk is assessed. Only patients with a low caries risk should be prescribed indirect restorations. Some of the more important caries risk factors are included in Table 1-1.

Table 1-1 **Caries risk factors**

Low caries risk	High caries risk
Minimally restored dentition	Heavily restored dentition
No history of replacement restorations	History of frequent restoration and re-restoration
Good oral hygiene	Poor oral hygiene
Exposure to topical fluoride in water, toothpaste or mouthwash	No exposure to topical fluoride
Diet: low frequency of sugar intake	Diet: frequent consumption of sugar
High socio-economic status	Low socio-economic status
No new carious lesions	Presence of new carious lesions

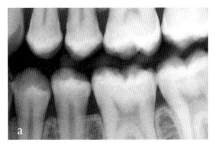 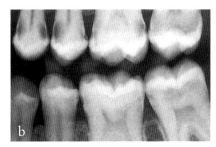

Fig 1-5 (a,b) A left bitewing radiograph of an 18-year-old patient (a), and four years later (b). This demonstrates that caries risk can change and the dentist should always be vigilant and continually assess risk. This patient's initial treatment should be pain relief, followed by a stabilisation phase and prevention. Indirect restorations should not be considered until successful prevention has been instituted and caries risk has been controlled.

Treatment Planning – Stabilisation and Prevention
For a patient with new and secondary caries (Fig 1-5a,b) it is important that treatment is carried out in phases. The first phase should address pain and other immediate problems. Thereafter, care should be aimed at prevention. This stage of treatment should include stabilisation of the lesions and protection with temporary and transitional restorations. This is necessary to ensure that extensive lesions do not progress during the preventive phase of treatment. It also allows a stepwise approach to caries removal.

Stepwise Excavation
In the tooth of a young patient with a relatively large pulp and a deep carious cavity, the risk of pulpal exposure during tooth preparation is high (Fig

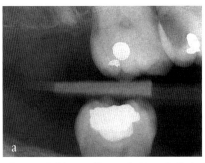 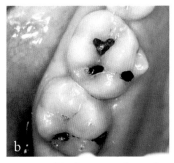

Fig 1-6 (a,b) A radiograph (a) and clinical appearance (b) of an extensive carious lesion on the distal aspect of the UR6 of a young teenage patient. In such a situation complete caries removal in one visit risks exposing the pulp. Stepwise excavation reduces this risk.

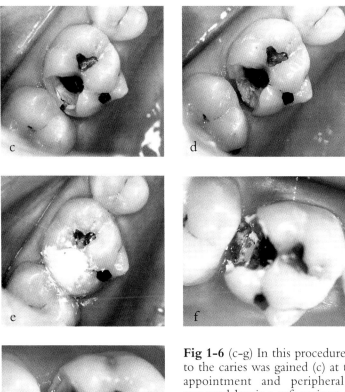

Fig 1-6 (c-g) In this procedure, access to the caries was gained (c) at the first appointment and peripheral caries removed leaving soft carious dentine pulpally (d). A provisional restoration was placed, using a polycarboxylate cement (e) and then left for 6 to 12 months. When the restoration was removed (f) and pulpal caries excavated no pulpal exposure occurred (g) (Series of images courtesy of Dr Nicola Innes).

1-6a-g). To avoid this, a stepwise approach to caries removal should be adopted, providing there are no signs or symptoms of pulpal pathology. Assessment should include a vitality or sensitivity test and a periapical radiograph of the tooth to ascertain if periradicular pathology is present.

During the initial stabilisation phase of treatment, access to carious dentine should be gained and peripheral caries at the enamel-dentine junction removed. This leaves soft carious dentine over the pulp, some of which can be excavated.

This is then covered with a setting calcium hydroxide lining material and the tooth restored with a composite, glass-ionomer or polycarboxylate cement provisional restoration. This provisional restoration should be left for six to twelve months, during which time bacteria within the lesion will become less metabolically active and reduce in number. This is because the intraoral source of sugar substrate has been blocked by the restoration, assuming a good peripheral seal. As the bacteria become less active, the lesion activity slows and may even stop, allowing time for pulp-dentine complex reactions to occur, in particular tubular sclerosis and reactionary dentine formation. When the six to twelve months has elapsed, reentry into the lesion allows further caries removal with a significantly reduced risk of pulpal exposure. This second stage of caries removal is best carried out when the patient is complying with dietary advice, and oral hygiene instruction has been shown to be satisfactory.

Caries Prevention
The preventive aspect of treatment should include disclosing of the teeth and oral hygiene instruction (Fig 1-7a,b). Plaque scores may be useful to demonstrate problem areas to the patient and to monitor patient compliance. Diet diaries should be filled in by the patient for three consecutive days, including two work days and one leisure day. This will allow cariogenic elements of the diet to be identified, including frequency of sugar intakes. Once these aspects of the diet have been highlighted in the diet diary, effective dietary advice can be given and topical fluoride should be prescribed.

Definitive Restorations

Once caries has been stabilised the next phase of the treatment can be considered, including decisions as to which teeth should be restored. Some teeth may

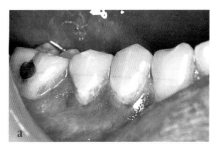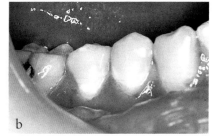

Fig 1-7 (a,b) Disclosing plaque allows plaque scores to be recorded. Monitoring oral hygiene over time allows patients to appreciate the association between the bacterial biofilm and the resultant caries when the plaque is partially (a) and completely removed (b).

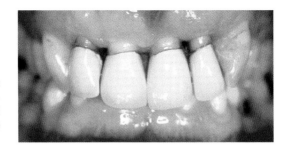

Fig 1-8 Gingival recession around upper incisor teeth following successful periodontal treatment subsequent to the placement of the crowns.

need extraction or root canal treatment. Initially, temporary restorations should be replaced with simple restorations. Before considering costly and time consuming indirect restorations, further assessment is required to ensure compliance with oral hygiene procedures and to assess caries activity. In this way, the success of primary preventive measures are reassessed, and only if they have been successful should indirect restorations be considered. If in doubt, further preventive advice is indicated, together with repeat follow-up reviews. Failure to do this is likely to result in a disastrous outcome as illustrated in Fig 1-4.

Periodontal Disease

Indirect restorations can fail as a result of periodontal disease. This can occur as a consequence of poor primary prevention prior to the placement of restorations. Aggravating factors such as overhanging margins and overcontoured crowns can lead to secondary failure. The patient in Fig 1-8 illustrates both of these points. Failure to establish good periodontal health prior to preparing the upper incisor teeth for crowns led to further attachment loss and recession. This was exacerbated by deficient crown margins. Successful periodontal treatment led to resolution of inflammation, further recession and the need for crown replacement to improve the appearance of the teeth.

A basic periodontal examination (BPE) should be carried out as part of the initial assessment. The examination is carried out by dividing the mouth into sextants: upper and lower left and right posterior; upper and lower anterior. A standard periodontal probe with a 0.5 mm ball end and a colour coded band from 3.5 to 5.5 mm should be used. The periodontal probe is "walked" around each tooth, examining at least six sites per tooth. For each sextant the highest score is recorded (Table 1-2).

Indirect restorations should not be considered until the treatment in Table 1-2 has been carried out, reevaluated and found to be successful. There

Table 1-2 **Basic periodontal examination and suggested treatment**

Periodontal (BPE) score	Definition	Suggested treatment
0	Healthy gingival tissue. No bleeding after gentle probing	No treatment
1	Coloured part of probe completely visible. No calculus or defective margins. Bleeding after gentle probing	Oral hygiene instruction only
2	Coloured part of probe completely visible. Supragingival calculus or defective margin of restoration	Oral hygiene instruction. Removal of calculus and correction of defective margins. Review in one year
3	Coloured part of probe enters periodontal pocket but remains partially visible	As for Code 2 but more time required. Plaque and bleeding scores at start and end of treatment. Probing depths at end of treatment. Repeat records after one year or less
4	Coloured part of probe completely disappears into pocket – probing depth ≥6 mm	Full probing depth chart (6 point pocket chart) required + gingival recession + furcation + intraoral radiograph of relevant teeth. As for 2. Root planing pockets >4 mm. Reexamine to assess results of periodontal treatment and whether further treatment required, possibly periodontal surgery
4★	★ denotes furcation involvement and/or attachment loss >7 mm	★ Specialist care required

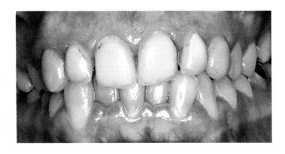

Fig 1-9 Poor gingival health at the time of placement of these composite vaneers compromised bonding leading to microleakage and staining of the restoration margins.

should be no signs of active periodontal disease in relation to the tooth being restored, such as bleeding on probing. Even gingival bleeding with a BPE score of 1 will make impression taking difficult and the resulting restoration is likely to have a poor fit. Consequently more plaque accumulation occurs and the disease process is perpetuated. Additionally, gingival inflammation at the time of placement will lead to bleeding and excess gingival crevicular fluid, which may compromise the cement lute. This predisposes to sensitivity, secondary caries and staining around tooth coloured restorations, including all-ceramic crowns and veneers (Fig 1-9).

If a new crown is required to replace an existing crown with a ledge or secondary caries, removal and initial replacement with a good fitting provisional restoration is necessary. This allows gingival health to be maintained prior to the definitive restoration. This is particularly important in relation to anterior teeth as resolution of gingival inflammation, let alone periodontal disease, typically leads to shrinkage of the tissues, exposing the crown margins. A definitive crown placed prior to resolving gingival and periodontal problems will lead to an unpredictable crown to gingival margin relationship.

Endodontic Failure

It is not uncommon to find evidence of periradicular pathology associated with teeth that have been crowned and from abutments for conventional bridgework. This may arise as a result of inadequate preoperative assessment, or as a direct consequence of the operative procedure.

Preoperative Assessment – Vitality Testing
Prior to considering an indirect restoration for a vital tooth, preoperative assessment should include testing of pulp vitality. Pulp vitality refers to a patent blood supply to a tooth. This can only be indirectly assessed by determining the neuronal response to various stimuli, thus the term sensitivity

testing is considered more appropriate. For teeth that have not been treated endodontically, this can conveniently be carried out by determining the pulpal response to thermal and electrical stimuli.

It is important when sensitivity tests are carried out that the tooth in question is isolated with cotton wool rolls and dried. This is particularly important when an electric pulp tester is used, as surface conduction in saliva to the gingival margin or adjacent teeth can lead to a false positive response. False positive responses can also be obtained in patients that are anxious with a heightened awareness and anticipation of pain and in multirooted teeth in which one or more canals may contain necrotic pulp tissue. After a tooth loses its blood supply and becomes non vital, C nerve fibres may remain capable of responding to stimuli for some time giving rise to a false positive response.

Likewise false negative responses are possible. Teeth in elderly patients and teeth which have been extensively restored may have significant deposits of normal physiological secondary dentine or tertiary dentine formation respectively giving a protective "insulating" effect. Following trauma a tooth may be concussed and whilst having a patent blood supply may not respond to stimuli for some time. Some patients' pain threshold may be high and they experience no pain from such stimuli.

The results of vitality or sensitivity testing can be unreliable and, as such, the results should not be taken in isolation. Other similarly sized and restored teeth should also be tested for comparisons and other tests such as percussion tests, a pain history and radiographic appearance should also be taken into account.

Restorative History of the Tooth

The restorative history of the tooth, in particular any history of pain, should be taken into account. With a history of repeated restoration and pain, the health of the pulp is likely to be compromised and further trauma from crown preparation may ultimately lead to the loss of vitality of the tooth.

It is also important to take into consideration any history of direct pulp capping. The literature demonstrating the success of direct pulp caps reports research carried out on teeth with a healthy pulp prior to trauma. In contrast, the long-term success of direct pulp capping in teeth that have suffered a carious exposure is relatively limited. This is particularly true in older teeth with more secondary and tertiary dentine or a reduced blood supply and limited healing potential. In these situations root canal treatment should be considered.

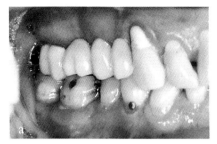 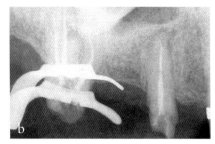

Fig 1-10 (a,b) Preparation of the UR5 and UR7 for metal-ceramic bridge retainers (a) has led to the loss of pulp vitality, necessitating the removal of the bridge and root canal treatment (b).

During tooth preparation, in particular crown preparation, pulpal damage is caused by heat generated between the bur and the tooth. The potential for such damage is greatest when preparing a tooth for a full coverage crown or bridge retainer (Fig 1-10a,b). This is because large amounts of tooth need to be removed to provide space for the metal and ceramic. To minimise such trauma tooth preparation should be carried out intermittently, with small amounts of tooth being removed at any one time and under copious water coolant.

When a tooth has lost vitality, subsequent to the placement of an indirect restoration, it is sometimes possible to carry out endodontic treatment through the restoration. This facilitates placement of a rubber dam and an aseptic technique, providing there is no secondary caries in relation to the restoration. However, access through a crowned tooth can be difficult because the original morphology of the tooth is lost. This can be made all the more difficult if significant amounts of tertiary dentine have formed prior to loss of vitality. Appearance may be impaired by shadows cast by metal crowns and amalgam cores. For these reasons, consideration should always be given to removing the crown prior to the endodontic treatment to decrease the risk of perforation (Fig 1-11).

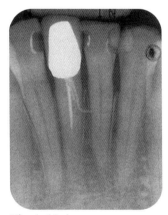

Fig 1-11 An attempt at root canal retreatment of LR1 through the metal-ceramic crown led to perforation as assessment of crown-root morphology was lost and vision difficult (Courtesy of Dr Carol Tait).

Aesthetic Failure

Failure to provide indirect restorations with a pleasing appearance compromises the clinical outcome. It is important that the patient's expectations are discussed and that the patient is aware of what may or may not be achievable in terms of aesthetics. In most cases a diagnostic wax-up is highly recommended, if not essential. Consider the patient in Fig 1-12 who has congenitally missing upper lateral incisor teeth and has recently lost the upper

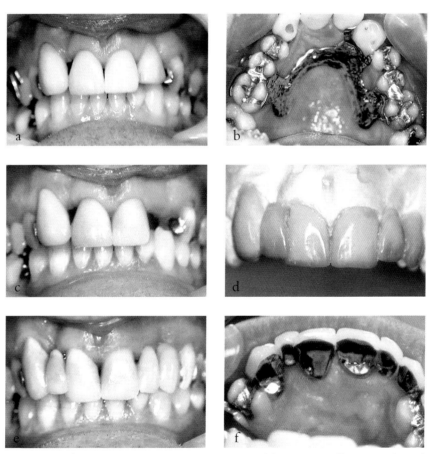

Fig 1-12 (a–f) In an attempt to close spaces created by congenitally missing lateral incisors and a missing upper canine, large crowns and an upper partial removable prosthesis were provided (a–c). The patient was unhappy with this appearance. This aesthetic failure could have been avoided if alternative diagnostic wax-ups were shown to the patient (d–f).

left canine. In an attempt to close the spaces between the teeth large crowns have been placed and the upper left canine replaced by means of a removable prosthesis. The patient was unhappy with the appearance of the crowns and the large interdental spaces. This costly exercise could have been avoided if the patient's expectations were realised with the aid of a diagnostic wax-up. In the case in question the patient was happy with smaller irregular teeth provided by a combination of crowns and bridges (Fig 1-12).

Mechanical Failure

Loss of Retention

Indirect restorations are luted with cement. Failure within the cement lute can lead to loss of the restoration. Various factors can influence the cement lute, including occlusal forces, tooth preparation, design and fit of the restoration, type of luting cement, and the cementation technique. Each of these factors is discussed in the subsequent chapters, but when decementation has occurred the reason should be determined, as failure to address the cause will lead to subsequent and repeated decementation.

Considerable attention is focussed on features of indirect restorations but it is retention or foundation work of the core which underpins the success of the restoration, which is why Chapter 3 has been devoted to this topic. The health of the dental pulp typically depends on the number of traumatic insults it has sustained, however, if any existing restoration, core or base in a tooth is suspect it must be removed. A previously placed core which appears to be caries free and well retained may not require replacement but, where there is doubt, it should be removed and replaced.

Catastrophic Fracture or Failure of Dental Material

Failure of the materials used for indirect restorations can result from inappropriate choice of materials, trauma or, more commonly, poor clinical and

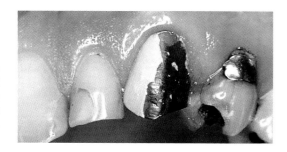

Fig 1-13 Poor laboratory technique and heavy occlusal loading in lateral excursion has led to fracture of the ceramic facing on this metal-ceramic crown.

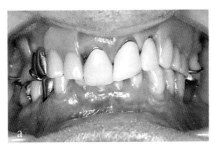 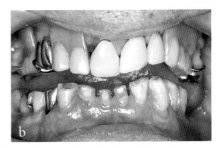

Fig 1-14 (a,b) Inappropriate extension of ceramic onto the palatal surface of crowns placed on the upper central incisor teeth has led to extensive wear of the lower incisor teeth.

laboratory techniques (Fig 1-13). As in all other aspects of restorative dentistry, techniques must be applied both appropriately and methodically, and all materials used strictly in accordance with the manufacturer's instructions.

Wear

Most indirect restorations resist wear, however, they can cause wear of the opposing teeth. Porcelain, especially when adjusted, damaged or worn can create excessive wear of opposing teeth (Fig 1-14) and as such should only be considered for the restoration of occlusal surfaces where appearance is of prime importance and there are no other signs of wear. If used to replace occlusal surfaces, porcelain must be carefully glazed or polished.

Fracture

Placing porcelain on the occlusal surface also increases the risk of fracture especially in patients with a parafunctional habit. If this is unavoidable, perhaps at a patient's insistence, and especially where numerous indirect restorations are concerned, consideration should be given to provision of a protective stabilisation splint to be worn at night time (see Chapters 7 and 8).

Frequently, cobalt chromium partial dentures are made in conjunction with crowns with rest seats as part of their design. It is important that these rest seats consist of metal, because porcelain ones cannot withstand the additional occlusal load and shear off (Fig 1-15). Full gold crowns or metal-ceramic crowns with metal occlusal surfaces should be chosen for this purpose. When providing crowns for partially dentate patients future dental treatment should be borne in mind. If a removable partial prosthesis will be provided at a latter date, study casts should be surveyed, a denture design completed and the

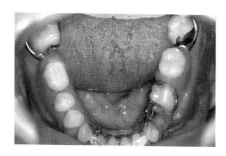

Fig 1-15 Use of ceramic on the mesial aspect of the crowns on the lower second molar teeth and rest seats for the removable cobalt chromium prosthesis has led to ceramic fracture.

appropriate rest seats, guide planes and undercuts incorporated into the crown (Fig 1-16a–g). This would have avoided the errors seen in the patient in Fig 1-15.

It is important that denture design is completed early in treatment planning, as this may influence tooth preparation. For example, where a rest seat is to be placed, occlusal reduction should be sufficient to accommodate the

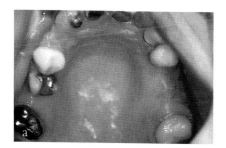
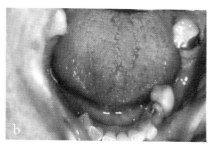
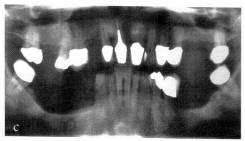
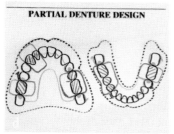

PARTIAL DENTURE DESIGN

Fig 1-16 (a–d) The partially edentulous patient seen in Fig 1-15. Following survey of the study casts the preliminary denture design for the lower arch was rejected (d) as a distobuccal undercut could not be created in the crowns on the molar teeth given the mesial inclination of these teeth, as seen in the dental panoramic tomogram (c).

15

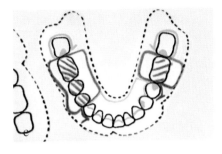
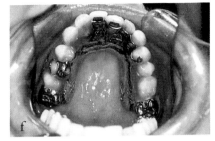
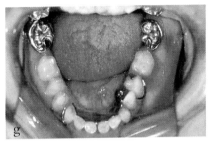

Fig 1-16 (e-g) An alternative design with circumferential clasps was possible (e) and appropriate rest seats, guide planes and undercuts were prescribed for the full veneer crowns on all four second molar teeth and metal-ceramic crown LL4 (f and g).

thickness of the crown and the rest seat. If this is not done, subsequent preparation of the crown for a rest seat may result in perforation.

Thorough examination, treatment planning and careful execution of procedures can prevent many of the failures seen in this chapter. The part played by prevention and postoperative monitoring cannot be over emphasised, especially when advanced restorations are planned. Failures will still occur, albeit less frequently, but when they do it is important that they are used to better understand ways to avoid any recurrence of the problem. Those who do not learn from failure are destined to encounter recurrence of their limitations.

Further Reading

Chapple ILC, Gilbert AD. Understanding periodontal diseases: assessment and diagnostic procedures in practice. Quintessentials Series. London: Quintessence Publishing Co. Ltd., 2002.

Kidd EAM. Essentials of Dental Caries. Oxford: Oxford University Press, 2005.

Rowe AH, Pitt Ford TR. The assessment of pulpal vitality. Int Endod J 1990;23:77-83.

Chapter 2
Indications for Crowns

Aim

To consider and review the indications for indirect full and partial coverage crowns.

Outcome

On reading this chapter the reader will appreciate the indications for crowns. The use of clinical examples helps the reader understand the complexities of the decision making process.

Introduction

The demand for crowns remains high. The development of new materials has, to some extent, reduced the need for full coverage restorations, but crowns will remain an important element of prosthodontics for decades to come. Crowns have various cost consequences, including the removal of large amounts of remaining tooth tissue. As a consequence the indications for crown placement need to be carefully considered. These indications are not definitive, remain largely subjective and typically have to be applied on a case by case assessment.

The indications for crowns are:
- replacement crowns
- protection of root-filled teeth
- broken down and worn teeth
- unsightly dental appearance
- cracked teeth
- realignment of occlusal plane.

Replacement Crowns

The most common indication for placing a crown in today's practice is the failure and replacement of an existing crown. On average crowns last 10 years, but under certain circumstances may remain in clinical service for 15–20 years. Various factors influence the longevity of crowns. These include caries, periodontal disease, loss of vitality, mechanical failure and changes to adjacent teeth with increasing age. The development of caries adjacent to the junction between tooth and crown remains one of the most common reasons for replacement, in particular, in older patients. Despite being a largely preventable disease as discussed in Chapter 1, caries remains the principle reason for both initial and replacement operative dentistry.

Apart from caries, mechanical and aesthetic failures are common indications for replacement crowns. Structural failure is a very obvious indication for replacement (Fig 2-1). Since porcelain is a brittle material, fractures are not uncommon, in particularly when the occlusal forces are high. This can be seen when opposing teeth contact the metal and porcelain junction on lateral and anterior guidance. The occlusal forces impact on this junction creating stress, which ultimately leads to fracture.

Another indication for replacement is an aesthetic failure. This may be clinical or laboratory failure or a consequence of the aging dentition. Bright or opaque crowns can be a result of insufficient depth reduction during crown preparation. Metal-ceramic crowns need 1.5–1.75 mm buccal reduction to provide sufficient space for the metal and porcelain. If this space is not provided opaque core porcelains used to hide the metal substructure make the crown appear bright or have a high value (Fig 2-2).

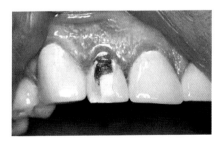

Fig 2-1 A common reason for the replacement of crowns is mechanical failure.

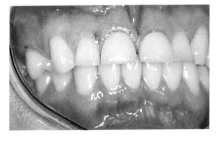

Fig 2-2 The two central incisors have a dull appearance and lack the natural translucency of teeth. The reason is that the preparation of the tooth created insufficient space for the metal and porcelain. There is insufficient space available for the aesthetic porcelains which are needed to hide the opaque inner ceramic core.

Fig 2-3 The appearance of long clinical crowns is difficult to mask. Once the length to width ratio exceeds 0.75–0.8 the appearance of the crowns is compromised. Replacement crowns are needed for this patient who already has long teeth. Increasing their length even further will accentuate the crown's height/width ratio and emphasise the black triangles between the teeth.

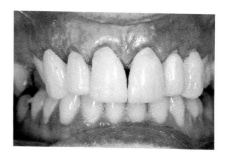

The problem with replacement crowns is that removal of caries and re-positioning of the gingival margin substantially reduces the amount of remaining tooth tissue. As the gingival margin migrates apically, the crown to root ratio is reduced and the clinical crown height is increased. Ideally, the width of the crown should be 0.75 to 0.85 of its length. Increasing the length beyond this ratio detracts from the aesthetic outcome giving what is commonly termed "tombstones" (Fig 2-3). Also as tooth length increases "black triangles" develop interdentally, compromising the dental appearance.

Long clinical crowns create a number of practical difficulties, not the least of which is tooth preparation. Avoiding undercuts on long preparations, let alone pulpal exposure, is difficult and can be avoided either by carefully controlling the taper of the preparation or by finishing the margin supragingivally. The latter has the disadvantage that a margin is visible above the gingival tissues and may be contraindicated in patients with a high lip line. Long clinical crowns can also appear unattractive.

Perhaps the most challenging clinical conundrum when replacing a crown is the position of the gingival margin. Subgingival margins create difficulties both in terms of recording an accurate impression and because patients have difficulty keeping the area plaque free (Fig 2-4). Both may increase the risk

Fig 2-4 The removal of the existing crown and caries has produced a deep subgingival distal margin. The decision as to whether the tooth justifies a crown is dependant on whether or not an accurate impression can be recorded along this margin. Crown lengthening would provide better access to the distal margin but will increase the cost.

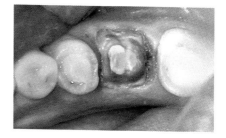

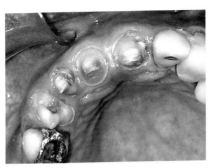

Fig 2-5 Replacement crowns on extensively restored upper anterior teeth. The teeth have had recurrent caries removed leaving preparations which are not ideal in shape for new crowns.

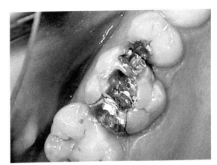

Fig 2-6 The loss of significant quantities of tooth during the access preparation and the provision of previous restorations has left the buccal and lingual walls weakened. In this case extracoronal protection with a crown or onlay is indicated.

of developing caries and periodontal disease along the margin. A common clinical dilemma is whether a crown is appropriate for an extensively restored tooth with a plastic restoration below the gingival margin. Placing expensive restorations on teeth with doubtful prognosis may lead to early failure. On the other hand weakened cusps are liable to fracture. With the increasing cost of materials and laboratory charges, the expectation of patients is that crowns should have a reasonable longevity, of around 10 years. If an accurate impression cannot be taken to ensure a good fit between crown and tooth the use of a crown to restore the tooth should be questioned. In some cases, however, a pragmatic approach can be justified provided the patient is fully informed of the alternatives and risks.

The other problem with replacement crowns is that the state of the underlying core is typically unknown prior to removal of the old crown. The core supporting the crown should have a near parallel taper approaching 15° with a form to maximise the retention and support of the crown. The collar of tooth remaining should be a minimum of 2 mm in height with near parallel preparation and a form which largely mirrors the anticipated shape of the crown. Once the old crown is removed it is not uncommon to find that the shape of the existing tooth preparation is far from ideal and not suited for its intended purpose (Fig 2-5). Removal of diseased dentine can further reduce the retention of a core and crown, leaving a choice between either electively root filling the tooth to gain additional retention or by relying on an adhesive luting cement.

Endodontically Treated Teeth

Not all root-filled teeth require an indirect coronal restoration. There is relatively little guidance in the literature as to which teeth require a crown following root treatment, as most research has been undertaken on extracted teeth. Traditional thinking is that root treated teeth are liable to fracture and therefore require occlusal coverage for protection. But this is not necessarily the case. A good guide is if the surface area of the access cavity exceeds one third of the occlusal surface of the tooth then a crown or onlay with cuspal coverage is justified (Fig 2-6). Similarly, if the lingual or buccal walls are undermined and the mesial and the distal marginal ridges are missing, protection by indirect restoration is advisable. The thinking that root-filled teeth become brittle through dehydration is tenuous. More likely, the removal of the roof of the pulpal chamber during access cavity preparation leaves the lingual and buccal walls weakened and unsupported, increasing the likelihood of fracture. Therefore, access preparation should be conservative, preserving wherever possible the mesial and distal surfaces of the tooth.

Extracoronal coverage with indirect restorations will provide protection to weakened and extensively prepared teeth. One of the most important preoperative assessments is the impact of any preparation upon the remaining tooth tissues and the core. For most plastic restorations, in particular amalgams, retention is dependent on the undercuts placed within the dentine walls. Removal of these undercuts during crown preparation will compromise the retention of the core, possibly necessitating an alternative restorative option.

Tooth Wear

Tooth wear tends to leave teeth with short clinical crowns (Fig 2-7). The common causes of tooth wear are erosion, attrition and abrasion – often in combination. Erosion is the loss of tooth structure from acids – commonly

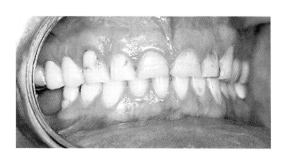

Fig 2-7 Short clinical crowns caused by tooth wear.

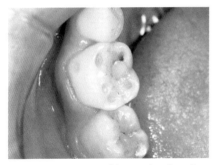

Fig 2-8a Erosion of the occlusal surface of a lower first molar. Dietary acids have eroded the occlusal surface exposing the dentine.

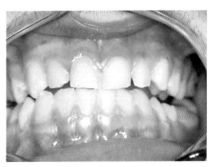

Fig 2-8b Erosion of the buccal surfaces by dietary acids has removed the enamel exposing the dentine. The appearance is smooth and shiny.

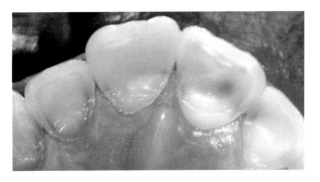

Fig 2-8c Gastric acids have eroded the palatal surfaces of the upper incisors exposing the dentine and almost the pulp.

dietary or gastric acids (Fig 2-8a-c). Attrition is the wear of tooth against tooth often associated with a parafunctional habit (Fig 2-9). Abrasion is the wear of teeth from non-tooth contacts such as toothbrushing or pen holding (Fig 2-10). Typically, the severe forms of erosion occur on the palatal surfaces of upper incisors and the occlusal surfaces of molar teeth. As the teeth become shorter compensatory mechanisms occur within the alveolar and gingival tissues to maintain a near normal vertical dimension. This increases the difficulty of restoring the teeth.

Erosion can be combined with bruxism making the provision of crowns more demanding. Parafunctional activity causing attrition creates particular restorative difficulties (Fig 2-9). The wear process leads to shortened teeth and the occlusal forces generated by the bruxing habit increase the risk of further damage to teeth and restorations. Porcelain materials are particularly susceptible to fracture from bruxing habits. Therefore, restoring worn teeth

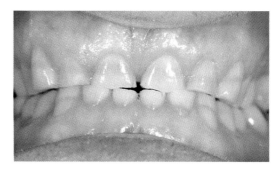

Fig 2-9 Bruxism causes tooth wear. The parafunctional habit will increase the loading on subsequent crowns increasing the risk of fracture of porcelain. Protection of the crowns with a full coverage hard acrylic splint will reduce the rate of wear.

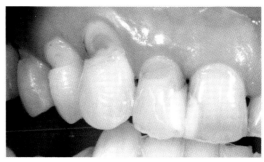

Fig 2-10 Abrasion and erosion of the buccal surfaces of the upper teeth associated with abrasion from toothbrushing and acids from the diet.

with crowns in patients with bruxism can lead to further problems including fracture of the restoration. In these circumstances it might be more prudent to protect the teeth from bruxism by prescribing full coverage hard acrylic night guards – Michigan splints. Alternatively, some operators suggest provision of canine risers to facilitate lateral guidance and reduce the impact of the damaging occlusal forces on the teeth.

In most cases tooth wear is a slow process. Monitoring tooth wear by comparing study casts over long periods of time can shed light on the aetiology of the condition, confirm that the wear is progressing slowly and reassure the patient. Restoring worn teeth with crowns, which are themselves liable to failure, may not preserve the longevity of the tooth. This is particularly important in young people in whom crowns may need to last many decades.

The indications for restoring worn teeth are as follows:
• uncontrolled tooth wear
• appearance
• uncontrolled sensitivity.

Many patients with tooth wear are concerned that the wear will result in the loss of their teeth later in life. For these patients dietary control, with management of reflux disease if indicated, might mean that the rate of tooth wear is reduced to such an extent that the life expectancy of the teeth matches that of the patient. However, in some instances the patient's concern for their dental appearance may justify operative intervention. This is despite the finding that once preventive advice has been given the rate of tooth wear often reduces to imperceptible levels. Wherever possible the cause of the wear should be diagnosed and preventive management commenced. For others, a specific diagnosis is not easily accomplished and treatment needs to be planned accordingly. The most important assessment in these circumstances is whether the severity of tooth wear justifies any restorative treatment. Mild to moderate tooth wear, where there is loss of enamel and dentine without significant loss of crown height, are appropriately managed by monitoring and preventive regimes. These regimes should include reduction in the consumption and frequency of dietary acids and the use of fluoride. Treatment of severe tooth wear will be partly influenced by the age of the patient and their ability to afford the cost of treatment. Crowns placed in young patients with severe wear will need repeated replacements over a lifetime and the patient needs to understand this risk. Situations involving short clinical crowns will be discussed later in Chapter 8.

On average composites used to treat tooth wear last 3–5 years and crowns may last around 10 years. With mild tooth wear in a young patient, composites might not last more than a few years. Once the restoration fails more tooth tissue will be removed when replacing the restoration. This starts the restorative cycle. Therefore, a longer term view would be to monitor the wear, as this might prolong the life of the tooth. Even with older patients having more severe wear the rate may not result in tooth loss during the patient's lifetime. The situation is less clear in younger patients with severe wear and middle-aged individuals with moderate to severe wear. In these situations the patient should be informed about the longevity of restorations, and the probability that progression of the tooth wear is slow, and given sufficient time to make an informed decision. The other major consideration is the cost of treatment because restorations for patients with tooth wear is expensive.

Despite tooth wear exposing significant areas of dentine, the development of sensitivity is uncommon on the palatal surfaces of upper incisors. On other tooth surfaces, in particular the cervical margins, sensitivity is more common and can indicate that the erosive component of the wear process is active.

Broken Down Teeth

The judgement as to when a restored tooth should be crowned is largely subjective. Many extensive amalgams and composite restorations remain serviceable for years with no detriment to the tooth. Improvements in materials and bonding techniques have reduced the need for extracoronal protection of weakened cusps. There is good evidence to suggest that well placed extensive amalgams or composites will last as long as crowns. But there are other examples where repeated fractures of extensively restored teeth necessitate coronal coverage with an indirect restoration. The difficulty is that there are few clinical signs to assist the clinician in deciding whether an extensively restored tooth needs a crown. To make the situation more difficult extensive restorations increase the complexity of designing a crown since the amount of unrestored enamel and dentine present may be limited. There is a body of opinion to say that the occlusion plays a part in the development of fractured teeth. If the occlusion is protected by canine guidance there is a possibility that on lateral excursions the occlusal surfaces of posterior teeth are protected from damaging lateral forces. These lateral forces may be associated with tooth or cusp fracture particularly when teeth are extensively restored. There is no consensus for this opinion, however, and the role of canine protection remains unproven.

Consider, for example an extensive amalgam with weakened buccal and lingual walls (Fig 2-11). The existing walls provide undercuts and are important in retaining the restoration. Removal of the walls during preparation of a full coverage crown results in loss of retention for the amalgam and will result in the loss of the core. Therefore, what might seem a straightforward decision to crown an extensively restored tooth may lead to problems of retaining the core.

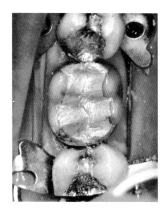

Fig 2-11 This extensive restoration relies on buccal and lingual walls for retention. If a crown is planned to protect the tooth the removal of the buccal and lingual walls to provide space for the crown may result in their removal and consequent loss of retention for the amalgam.

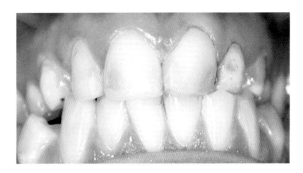

Fig 2-12 These extensive composites were placed five years ago and have been maintained by periodical refinishing. The composites have been a good alternative to crowns.

This problem may be overcome by choosing an intracoronal restoration made in gold or porcelain and so preserve the weakened cuspal walls.

Appearance

A commonly cited reason for placing a crown is to improve the appearance of the tooth, in particular an anterior tooth. Modern aesthetic composites combined with reliable dentine bonding agents produce a good long-lasting restoration (Fig 2-12). The need therefore, to crown teeth with extensive composites may be limited. The advantage of composites is that part of the natural translucence of the tooth is preserved, in particular along the cervical margin. It is in this area, at the crown to tooth margin, that the appearance of most crowns is compromised. Although crowns can appear natural they often lack the natural vibrancy or translucency of natural teeth.

A crown consists of an inner layer of metal or high strength porcelain which is opaque and prevents light transmission. This inner non-reflective surface needs to be masked by aesthetic porcelains. Around the occlusal/incisal surfaces the translucency of the crown can be enhanced by layering aesthetic

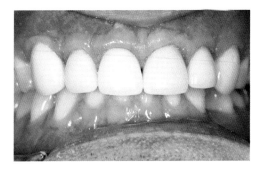

Fig 2-13 The metal-ceramic crowns have reasonable incisal translucency but along the cervical margin the opacity of the underlying metal results in an obvious colour change. Even cutting back the metal along this margin and finishing in porcelain may result in abrupt colour change and make the appearance of crowns more noticeable.

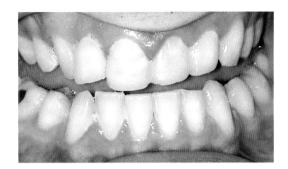

Fig 2-14 These composites required replacement with crowns as their appearance was no longer acceptable to the patient.

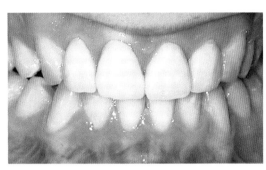

Fig 2-15 The replacement crowns improved the appearance of the teeth.

porcelains, but this is not possible at the gingival margin. At this junction the differences between the light transmission through the tooth and through the crown is particularly noticeable and this is where most crowns fail to match the adjacent natural teeth (Fig 2-13). Although all-ceramic crowns can to some extent overcome these deficiencies, compared with metal fused to porcelain crowns, they require substantial tooth removal to achieve this appearance. Therefore, although crowns can be made to appear natural, they have limitations. Despite these limitations and the qualities of modern composite materials, the need for crowns to improve the appearance of unsightly teeth remains a part of everyday practice (Fig 2-14 and Fig 2-15).

Cracked Teeth

Teeth commonly include fracture lines or visible cracks but only rarely do they produce symptoms (Fig 2-16). Once symptoms develop, however, a coronal coverage restoration is often indicated. Diagnosing cracked cusps or teeth can be difficult. Normally, pain starts on biting or on the release of the biting load. It is instant and poorly localised. It can affect both unrestored or restored teeth.

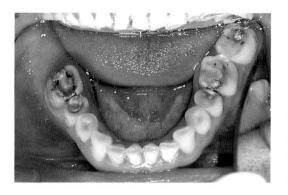

Fig 2-16 Cracked teeth can be difficult to diagnose. Occasionally, a crack or fracture line is visible on the crown but often the symptoms produced on biting, which are relieved immediately after occluding, are the only reliable sign.

Large extensive restorations in teeth with visible cracks together with the presence of symptoms can be diagnostic. Some assistance can be obtained by applying firm pressure through a probe handle onto the suspect cusp to illicit pain. Alternatively, a cotton wool roll, a piece of rubber dam, wooden wedge or a tooth sleuth can be placed between the teeth on the suspected area and the patient asked to bite together. The extent of the crack can also be highlighted with disclosing solution (Fig 2-17a and 2-17b).

Unfortunately, if the crack is allowed to progress the pulp may become involved and in certain cases the tooth splits. Therefore, occlusal protection is needed with either a full or partial coverage indirect restoration, most commonly of gold. A periapical radiograph and vitality test should be performed to assess pulpal status.

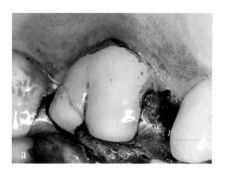 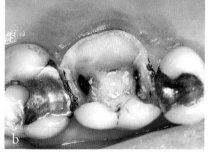

Fig 2-17 Disclosing solution has been used to highlight the crack along the palatal wall. The crack has been propagated resulting in the fracture of the palatal cusp. The remaining tooth structure, although weakened, is restorable.

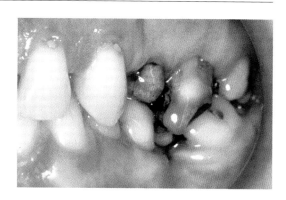

Fig 2-18 Overerupted teeth may need a crown to create interocclusal space for an opposing tooth.

Realignment of the Occlusal Plane

There are few indications for crowns to improve the occlusal plane. One example is the overeruption of teeth or cusps which interfere with the provision of restorations in the opposing arch (Fig 2-18). Occasionally, occlusal adjustment is sufficient to create the necessary space but once significant areas of dentine are exposed a crown is indicated.

Further Reading

Bartlett D, Brunton PA. Aesthetic Dentistry. Quintessentials Series. London: Quintessence Publishing Co. Ltd., 2005.

Hawthorne WS, Smales RJ. Factors influencing long-term restoration survival in three private dental practices in Adelaide. Aus Dent J 1997;42:59-63.

O'Sullivan M. Fixed prosthodontics. Quintessentials Series. London: Quintessence Publishing Co. Ltd., 2005.

Smith BGN. Planning and making crowns and bridges. London: Martin Dunitz, 1998.

Stoll, R, Sieweke M, Pieper K, Stachniss V, Schulte A. Longevity of cast gold inlays and partial crowns – a retrospective study at a dental school clinic. Clin Oral Investig 1999;3:100-104.

Wagner J, Hiller KA, Schmalz G. Long-term clinical performance and longevity of gold alloy vs. ceramic partial crowns. Clin Oral Investig 2003;7:80-85.

Walton TR. A 10-year longitudinal study of fixed prosthodontics: clinical characteristics and outcome of single-unit metal-ceramic crowns. Int J Prosthodont 1999;12:519-526.

Chapter 3
Retention of Cores

Aim

The aim of this chapter is to familiarise the reader with the need to place reliable, retentive cores.

Outcome

On reading this chapter the reader should understand the importance of cores for vital and non-vital teeth.

Introduction

The most commonly placed indirect restoration is a full coverage crown. The reason for the placement of such a restoration is usually a badly broken down, worn or heavily restored tooth. In these situations the cavity is often unretentive and the remaining tooth tissue weak and thin. During crown preparation the remaining tooth tissue is further reduced. The retention of the core therefore underpins the ultimate success of the indirect restoration. How this retention is achieved will depend on the vitality of the tooth and the type of core material, which in turn will be dictated by the type of crown and the particular circumstances.

Vital Teeth

The ideal root canal filling is a vital healthy pulp, which should be preserved wherever possible. Retention for a core can be achieved using dentine adhesives, slots and grooves and with increasing infrequency dentine pins. In extreme situations, elective endodontic treatment may be needed to utilise the pulp chamber or root canal space for a crown.

Dentine Adhesives

Dentine bonding agents have improved dramatically over the last two decades and are now reliable for bonding composite and ceramics to tooth tissues. There is no evidence that an amalgam core will perform better than one of composite. One of the advantages of composite over amalgam for a core is that the

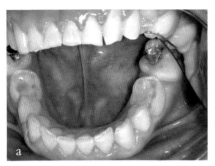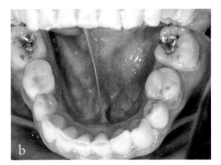

Fig 3-1 (a,b) Composite cores placed on retained deciduous molars in preparation for metal-ceramic crowns.

material reliably bonds to the tooth, it can be prepared immediately and conserves tooth tissue as undercuts are not required for retention.

Composite Cores

There is no alternative to composite on anterior teeth, whereas posteriorly the choice between composite and amalgam is more balanced. Whatever material is chosen, there should be sufficient tooth tissue remaining to retain the core. Although bond strengths between dentine adhesives and dentine approach that of enamel, caution is needed if the bond is the major component of retention for a core. If insufficient tooth tissue remains, either crown lengthening can be used to surgically lengthen the tooth, or in extreme situations elective root treatment may be required. Occasionally, in patients with canine guidance, where on lateral excursions the molar/premolars have limited, if any, contact, direct bonding of a crown to a flattened tooth surface is possible (Fig 3-1). More commonly direct composites can be placed with the aid of an adhesive to form a core (Fig 3-2).

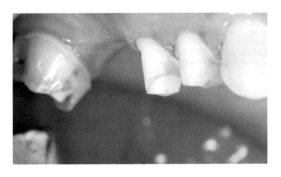

Fig 3-2 Composite cores placed on upper premolar teeth and prepared for a metal-ceramic crown and bridge retainer.

Some manufacturers have produced bespoke fibre reinforced core materials. These materials are high strength materials which have a consistency similar to natural teeth when prepared. In addition, they come together with plastic core formers made to the ideal taper and shape of a preparation. These materials are dual cured and packaged with the appropriate dentine bonding agent.

Glass-ionomer Cores

There are few indications for using glass-ionomers for cores in anterior or posterior teeth. One limited example is small additions to existing cores which have fractures involving only part of a cusp. The bond strength between a glass-ionomer cement and tooth or existing restoration is weaker than that of bonded composite, and the potential for loss of the addition increases as the amount of the material increases. Extensive additions may result in the loss of the glass-ionomer cement during a later stage in the provision of the crown. Sometimes it is worthwhile including the fractured portion in the preparation or completely removing the intracoronal part of the restoration. This is especially useful in teeth with short clinical crowns (Fig 3-3a,b).

Amalgam Cores

Amalgam remains a useful material for cores, but has the disadvantage that it does not bond to tooth tissue (Fig 3-4). To overcome this, a number of materials have been used to bond amalgam to tooth tissue including 4-META resins and BIS-GMA adhesive cements. Ideally, the adhesive resin cement

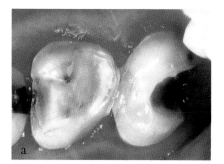 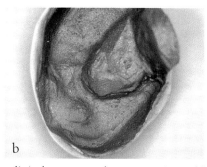

Fig 3-3 (a,b) These molar teeth have short clinical crowns and are to receive gold crowns/onlays as part of a complex treatment plan. Additional retention can be gained by removing the conventional restorations, blocking out undercuts with composite and utilising the intracoronal element in the preparation (a). The fit surface of the casting for the second molar tooth can be seen (b).

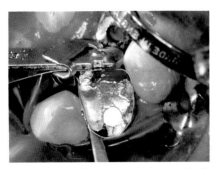

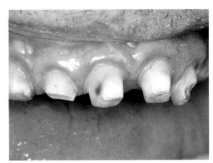

Fig 3-4 Amalgam core being packed. Minimum tooth tissue will remain after crown preparation, necessitating bonding of the amalgam.

Fig 3-5 The short clinical crown of the upper right lateral incisor has led to an unretentive crown preparation. Buccal and proximal slots have been cut to improve retention.

should be chemically or dual cured. The resin is thinly coated onto the cavity walls and the amalgam is packed directly onto it before it sets. Laboratory studies indicate that the retention provided by bonded amalgams is equal to or greater than undercuts grooves, dovetails or pins. Other laboratory and clinical studies suggest that bonded amalgams reduce leakage and postoperative sensitivity. On balance, bonded amalgams should be considered in preference to the placement of pins.

Slots and Grooves

Undercuts, slots and grooves can be cut into the remaining dentine and may be found to enhance retention and resistance form to a greater extent than dentine pins. They have the advantage over dentine pins that there is no potential for inadvertent placement of a pin into the pulp or periodontal ligament or loosening or exposure of the pin during carving. On balance they should be used in preference to pins wherever possible. In Fig 3-5, the slots cut labially and proximally increase the surface area over the preparation, help resist unseating occlusal forces and reduce the taper between opposing walls of the preparation.

Dentine Pins

Pin Types

Self-tapping pins have a diameter larger than the drill and are more commonly used (Fig 3-6). However, the advent of reliable resin adhesive luting cements has led to their demise. Historically, cemented pin systems involved

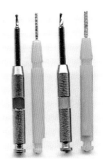

Fig 3-6 Two sizes of a self-tapping pin system (Stabilok, Fairfax Dental, UK), showing pin drill and corresponding self-shearing pin.

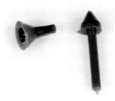

Fig 3-7 Plastic burn out pins that can be incorporated into the wax pattern of crowns or onlays during construction.

a drill slightly larger than the diameter of the pin which was cemented into the prepared pin hole, and friction retained pins were driven into pin channels of slightly smaller diameter than the pin. Passively fitting pins were also used in indirect castings when conventional retention was poor (Fig 3-7).

Pins are usually placed in the region of a missing cusp, 1.0–1.5 mm in from the external surface to avoid furcation areas. This location usually corresponds to the safest place for pin placement and allows adequate bulk of restorative material to be packed around the pin. Once the position has been chosen, the dentine forming the floor of the cavity should be flattened. In addition, a small round bur can be used to create a dimple in the dentine at the insertion site to reduce the risk of the pin drill being displaced from skating around on the dentine (Fig 3-8a-e). The twist drill should be aligned with the root surface prior to preparation to determine the correct angulation of the drill. Maintaining the same angulation, the drill is moved to the dimple and the pin hole prepared with single vertical plunge (a definite in-out movement). The pin drill should be inserted to its full extent of the shoulder and a speed reducing handpiece used to reduce the amount of heat generated. The pin is then inserted and once at its full depth it automatically shears. The pin can be bent towards the middle of the tooth to stay within the contour of the core.

To achieve success the following should be followed as a guide:
• Depth of the pin in dentine should be 2–2.5 mm.

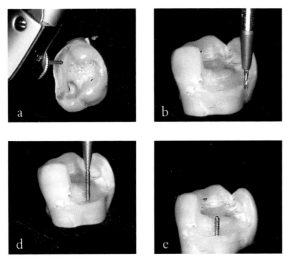

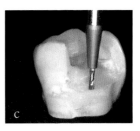

Fig 3-8 (a-e) Technique for placement of a self-threading, self-shearing pin. A dimple is cut onto a flat surface of dentine away from any furcation areas (a), the pin drill is aligned with the outer surface of the tooth (b), without altering the angulation it is brought to the dimple (c) and the pin hole is cut. The pin is then "threaded" into this hole (d) and automatically shears when it reaches the base (e) (Courtesy of Professor A Grieve).

- Depth of pin in restorative material should be 2–2.5 mm.
- At least 1 mm of core material should surround the pin.
- Pin placement should be at least 0.5 mm inside the enamel-dentine junction.

The first two points ensures optimum retention within the dentine and the restorative material. Pins only serve to retain the core and do not add strength or support the restorative material. In fact the converse is true, pins act as a line of weakness within the restorative material, which is particularly pronounced in amalgam. Consequently, an adequate amount of material should surround the pin. This is a dilemma when pins are used to retain cores for metal-ceramic crowns. Consider the situation in Fig 3-9 where a clear core form has been placed to allow a buccal shoulder preparation. Little or no core material is likely to surround the pin. The only solution is to place the pin further pulpally, increasing the risk of perforation into the pulp. In this situation an alternative to pins should be considered.

There are a number of disadvantages associated with dentine pins:
- They induce stresses within the dentine.
- They cause dentinal crazing.
- Self-shearing pins may fail to penetrate to the full depth of the pin hole.

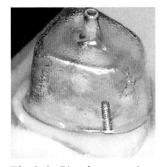

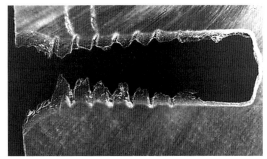

Fig 3-9 Pin placement in a position to avoid pulp perforation leaves inadequate space for core placement, as seen through a clear core former.

Fig 3-10 This micrograph shows cracks forming in dentine in relation to the threads of the pin (Courtesy of Professor A Grieve).

- The fracture resistance of core materials is reduced, particularly with amalgam, as the number of pins increases.
- Perforation into the periodontium and pulp (if vital) can occur.

Because the diameter of the pin thread is wider than the diameter of the hole cut, distortion of the dentine is inevitable and this leads to crazing of the dentine (Fig 3-10). If pins are placed too close to the enamel-dentine junction, this distortion can lead to enamel fracture and if the pins are placed too close together communication of the lateral crazing can lead to failure. On insertion, the frictional forces increase as more of the pin engages the dentine and frequently the pins shear off before penetrating the full depth of the pin hole (Fig 3-11). When this occurs, a gap of between 0.5 mm and 0.75 mm remains at the bottom of the pin hole. Whilst this seems small it represents a 25% to 33% discrepancy for a 2 mm to 2.5 mm pin. This leads

Fig 3-11 This pin has sheared off before reaching the full depth of the pin hole (Courtesy of Professor A Grieve).

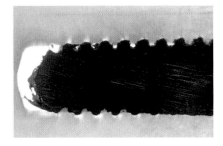

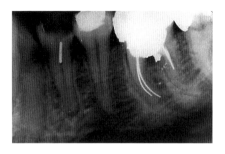

Fig 3-12 Periapical radiograph showing pin perforation into the pulp chamber.

to decreased retention and a pin that is too long within the cavity which typically interferes with the occlusion and strength of the core material.

Most problems with pin placement involve perforation into the pulp and periodontium. Complete perforation of the pin into the pulp is obvious (Fig 3-12) and requires removal of the pin and root canal treatment. Partial perforation into the pulp may not be so obvious clinically and the incidence of this has been estimated at about 30%. This may result in postoperative sensitivity but it may not become apparent clinically until loss of pulp vitality occurs. Perforation into the periodontium is far more obvious clinically (Fig 3-13a,b) and if not removed can lead to chronic periodontal problems and angular bony defects. This occurs more commonly in tilted or angulated teeth and can be avoided if a radiograph is used preoperatively to assess the tooth and the pin drill aligned with the root surface.

It is clear that whilst dentine pins have been an important inclusion in the dental armamentarium for retention of restorations, their disadvantages

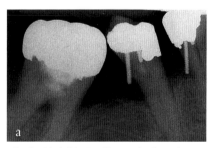 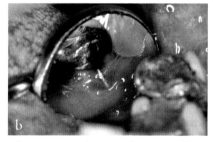

Fig 3-13 (a,b) Radiograph showing pin perforation into the periodontium of two premolar teeth and resultant periodontal angular bony defects (a). Pin perforation into the periodontium is not always evident clinically, unlike the case in this lower second molar tooth (b).

should be sufficient to discourage their routine use. Alternatives to achieve adequate retention should therefore be considered.

Non-vital and Endodontically Treated Teeth

The process of root treating a tooth removes significant tooth tissue and increases the risk of subsequent fracture. An early suggestion for this increased risk of fracture was the result of loss of moisture following the loss of vitality of the pulp. The most likely cause however, is the loss of extensive tooth tissue needed to gain access to the root canals. Specifically, it is the loss of the cuspal inner slopes during access preparation that reduces the capacity of the tooth to resist deformation.

There are few long-term well conducted investigations into the indications for crowns for endodontically treated teeth. One of the largest studies by Sorensen and Martinoff (1984) examined 1273 endodontically treated teeth over a period of 25 years. The authors reported that crowns on upper and lower endodontically treated incisors did not significantly increase clinical success. It was reported, however, that crowns on maxillary premolar and molar teeth improved survival rates. The finding was similar for mandibular teeth. Similar reviews by others have confirmed the finding.

In certain situations where there is extensive loss of tooth tissue elective endodontics may be indicated to enable the pulp chamber or root canal to aid core retention. Typically, this occurs in extensively restored anterior teeth with little supragingival tooth structure remaining. In this situation, the success rate of the endodontics is normally high, assuming all the vital pulp tissue is removed and the root filled using accepted endodontic techniques.

Posterior Teeth

Posts are generally unnecessary in posterior teeth. Moderately sized access cavities normally allow the utilisation of the pulp space to provide retention for the core. The presence of undercuts within the remaining walls and the roots can provide adequate retention and strength to the core (Fig 3-14a,b). Post placement in these situations weakens the tooth further and because the roots are often thin and curved, root perforation is a significant risk.

When a molar tooth has been root treated, it is important to remove all the gutta percha from the pulp chamber leaving well defined gutta percha stumps (Fig 3-15a). The pulp chamber can then be assessed for undercuts.

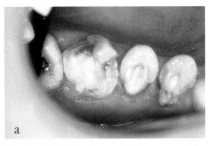
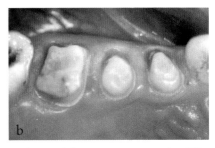

Fig 3-14 (a,b) Root-filled upper right premolars and first permanent molar. The gutta percha stumps have been covered with a resin-modified glass-ionomer lining material. Retention in the remaining chamber (a), together with the use of a dentine bonding agent will be sufficient to retain composite cores (b).

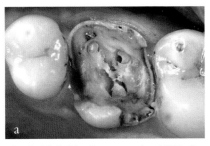
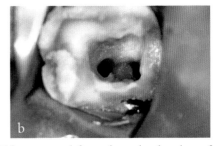

Fig 3-15 (a,b) Gutta percha (GP) should be removed from the pulp chamber of root-filled teeth leaving only GP stumps visible (a). Where inadequate retention for the core is obtained from the pulp chamber, 3 mm of GP can be removed from the entrance of the root canal (b) – the Nayyar core.

If not undercut, gutta percha can be removed from the coronal 3 mm of the root canal and the core material packed into the entrance to the root canals (Fig 3-15b). Because the root canals usually diverge, sufficient undercut will be obtained for retention. This technique has been referred to as a Nayyar core.

If the pulp chamber is sufficiently undercut for retention further gutta percha removal is unnecessary. In these situations the floor of the pulp chamber should be covered with a resin-modified glass-ionomer (Fig 3-14a). This provides an additional coronal seal for the root canal system and any accessory canals in the furcation area. Consideration should be given to a resin-based material with an appreciable shade mismatch with the remaining tooth tissue, if root canal retreatment is necessary. If amalgam is used, consideration should be given to amalgam bonding to facilitate an improved coronal seal.

Anterior and Single Rooted Teeth

Teeth that have been root filled as a result of trauma, and have most of the coronal tooth tissue remaining, do not normally require crown placement, because they are no more susceptible to fracture than intact teeth. Small fractures can be restored by simple composite restorations. The majority of root-filled teeth will however, have suffered significant loss of coronal tooth tissue, usually as a result of caries and restorative procedures. Nayyar cores are not normally used for anterior teeth because the pulp chambers are smaller and an alternative approach to core retention is required. Posts normally provide the solution.

Post Space Preparation

There are a considerable number of post systems available, but the requirements of root filling removal and post space preparation remain the same for anterior teeth. In most situations, post space preparation can be carried out at the time of obturation. This has the advantage that the operator is familiar with the root canal morphology, working length and there is no risk of losing the reference point from where the working length was measured, due to loss of tooth tissue or restoration between appointments.

The definitive post should be cemented as soon as possible as the creation of a good coronal seal to the root canal system is recognised as critical to the success of the endodontic treatment. Many dentists will be cautious of this as they would wish to be sure of the success of the endodontic treatment first. In most situations this is not necessary as the success rates of endodontic treatment has been recorded to be as high as 96%. There are a number of factors which influence endodontic success:
- rubber dam
- an aseptic technique
- copious irrigation with sodium hypochlorite
- good root canal preparation and obturation.

If root canal preparation is accompanied by complete removal of the remaining vital pulp tissue and there is no evidence of periradicular pathology or symptoms throughout treatment, success is normally ensured. A period of postoperative monitoring should be considered in situations where a heavily infected necrotic pulp is removed, where there is evidence of periradicular pathology, and where there have been symptoms throughout treatment. This, however, should be kept as short as possible, as temporary post crowns provide inadequate coronal seal and have a tendency to fail.

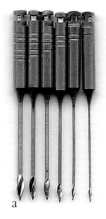 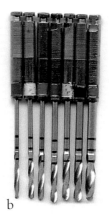

Fig 3-16 (a,b) Non end-cutting Gates Glidden burs for gutta percha removal (a) and ParaPost (Coltène Whaledent Ltd) twist drills for post space preparation (b). Note: always use smallest bur in sequence and work up incrementally through the sizes until the desired diameter is reached.

Root filling material, typically gutta percha, should be removed with a non-end cutting bur such as Gates Glidden (SuperDent, Switzerland) (Fig 3-16a). The smallest bur should be used first, working up through the sizes until size 3 or 4 is reached. The smallest post space drill from the post system chosen can then be used (Fig 3-16b), again working up through the series of sizes until the desired diameter post is reached. Working systematically through the increasing sizes of rotary instruments has a number of advantages. It ensures symmetrical post space preparation around the root canal and reduces weakening of the root and the risk of perforation (Fig 3-17). It also reduces the amount of heat generated which, if not controlled, may damage periodontal ligament cells, as smaller amounts of material or tooth tissue are removed at a time. Heat can also be used to remove the gutta percha. A measured System B plugger (Analytic Technology, Redmond, USA) is ideal for this. Chemicals such as chloroform and oil of turpentine have also been used; however, whilst useful in removing gutta percha for root canal retreatment

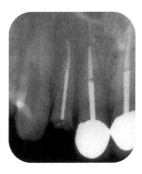

Fig 3-17 Periapical radiograph showing root-filled upper incisor teeth and ideal post space preparation, leaving approximately 4 mm of gutta percha apically. The narrower post in the lateral incisor has fractured.

Fig 3-18 Upper anterior teeth prepared for crowns. The upper left central incisor and upper right lateral incisor have cast post and cores cemented. The upper right lateral incisor has no coronal tooth tissue present and hence no ferrule. The upper left central incisor has approximately 1 mm of coronal tooth tissue present, sufficient for a small ferrule effect when the crown is cemented.

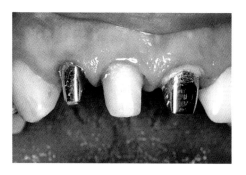

cases, the use of such chemicals is not advocated for post space preparation, as there is no control over the depth of softening of the gutta percha.

Ideally, to maintain an adequate apical seal, 4–5 mm of well condensed gutta percha should remain in the root end (Fig 3-17). Without compromising the apical seal, the length of the post should be at least the length of the clinical crown and preferably longer. This is critical for adequate retention. Post diameter has been shown to have relatively little effect on retention. The diameter of the post at the apical extreme should not exceed one third of the diameter of the root at the same level. A post that is too wide apically leads to a weakened root and has an increased risk of root fracture. It is also important to preserve as much coronal tooth tissue as possible as the length of tooth tissue braced by the crown (the ferrule effect) significantly reduces the risk of vertical root fracture (Fig 3-18). The retention of crowns relying on posts for retention is greatly improved by utilising the remaining coronal tooth tissue surrounding the post hole. A ferrule provides important bracing against lateral forces impacting upon the crown.

Choice of Post

The choice of which post to use is confusing, because there are many types available commercially. Indirect metal posts, that are cast as post and cores in the laboratory are commonly used, and if made well have been shown to be successful in clinical practice (Fig 3-19a,b and Fig 3-20a-c). The cast post however, suffers from a number of drawbacks. These include:

- It is frequently short leaving a void between the post tip and the root filling.
- Castings can have porosities at the junction of the core and post leading to post fracture.
- The crown needs to be made using a separate impression of the cemented

43

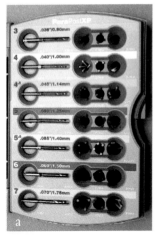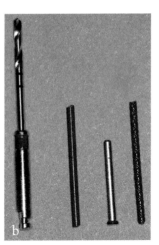

Fig 3-19 (a,b) ParaPost XP System (Coltène Whaledent Ltd) used for making cast post and cores (a). Taking the red (1.25 mm) post as an example (b): from left to right, the post preparation drill, smooth sided plastic impression post, the titanium temporary post and the serrated plastic burn out post, which the technician inserts into the casting of the post hole and onto which he or she waxes up the core, ready for casting using the lost wax technique.

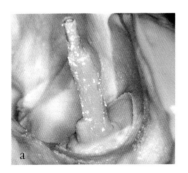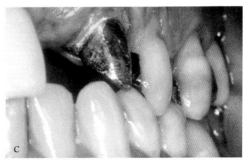

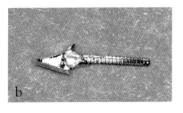

Fig 3-20 (a-c) A putty and wash impression of a post space preparation for a cast post and core in an upper left canine (a). The wash has been syringed around the root face and the impression post has been inserted through the wash, dragging it into the post hole, giving an impression of the irregular post preparation. Note that an antirotational groove has been cut, however this is unnecessary if sufficient coronal tooth tissue remains for a ferrule. A different cast post and core prior to cementation (b). Cemented cast post and core for the patient seen in (a), ready for a second impression for a metal-ceramic crown (c).

post and core. This adds greatly to chair-side time and the cost of providing a crown.

• Finally, being metal a cast post is unsuitable for use under tooth coloured crowns.

The main indications for cast post and cores are for irregularly shaped canals where the use of preformed posts is contraindicated and where the angulation of the core needs to be different from the long axis of the root.

An alternative to an indirect post is the use of preformed post systems. There is an extensive range of preformed post systems varying from tapered, parallel, threaded to non-threaded or combination systems. Active posts engage the dentine by a thread, whilst passive posts rely on the cement lute for primary retention. In general, parallel sided posts are more retentive than tapered posts, and threaded posts are more retentive than serrated posts, which in turn are more retentive than smooth sided posts. Whichever post system is used, the length of the post is one of the most critical factors. Serrated posts improve the flow of cement along the dentine walls increasing retention. Active posts should also be cemented in place so as to gain secondary retention and more importantly to achieve a good coronal seal. All post systems if used properly, have sufficient retention, therefore selection should be based on the system least likely to cause fracture in clinical service.

A preoperative periapical radiograph is indicated to assess the diameter of the root at the apical extent of the post. Preoperative radiographs are invaluable, but it is important to appreciate that the radiograph is a 2D image, and that some teeth have roots with a figure of eight shape when cut in cross section. Particular care should be taken over teeth which have very narrow root canals, notably lower incisors and upper second premolars with single roots.

Threaded posts should be used only when retention is compromised. This is usually necessary when a post is needed for a short or curved root. The threads have a wider diameter than the prepared post hole and as such introduce stresses into the remaining dentine. The counter threads cut into dentine, on the internal aspect of the post hole, and can either be created at the time of post insertion (self-threading) (Fig 3-21) or can be cut prior to post cementation (pretapped) (Fig 3-22a,b). In theory, the latter introduce less stress into the dentine as the post threads follow the pretapped counter threads on insertion, with minimal distortion of the dentine. Tapered threaded posts systems should be avoided as there is a combined wedging effect in addition

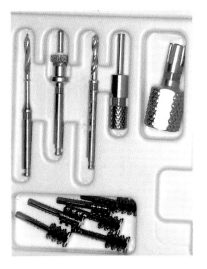

Fig 3-21 Radix anchor post system, consisting of: from left to right, a reamer to remove gutta percha, a diamond coated root facer used to produce a flat surface onto which to seat the post head, a parallel sided post preparation drill, a gauge to check the seat of the post and orientation of the post preparation, the post driver, and at the bottom the threaded Radix anchor posts. The post is self threading and should be used carefully. The post is gradually introduced into the post hole turning clockwise allowing the post to cut the dentine in stages. After each full turn remove the post, wash and irrigate the root canal and then reinsert the post. Continue preparing the post hole until the full length is inserted into the canal.

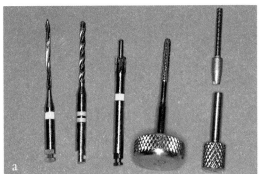
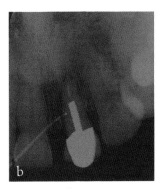

Fig 3-22 (a,b) K4 Anchor system: from left to right, reamer used to remove gutta percha, parallel post space drill, root facer used to flatten the root face to stabilise the head of the post, a tapping device (thread cutter) and post ready to be inserted into its driver (a). Radiograph showing a Kurer Anchor post in situ (b). The use of root facers has the disadvantage of removing valuable coronal tooth tissue and hence eliminating the ferrule effect. This together with the stresses induced by the threads has led to root fracture and sinus formation. A gutta percha point has been inserted into the sinus prior to taking the radiograph.

to these stresses (Fig 3-23a,b). In an attempt to overcome these problems a split post was created, the Flexi Post (Fig 3-24), which collapses when inserted into the prepared post hole. It is thought by some clinicians that the need for threaded posts has been superseded by resin adhesive luting cements. It should be remembered, however, that posts cemented with adhesive lut-

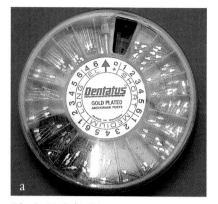
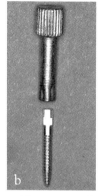

Fig 3-23 (a,b) Dentatus screw post system (a), an example of a tapered threaded post. A post is seen with its driver ready to be attached (b).

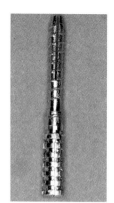

Fig 3-24 Flexi Post with split end.

ing cements may prove difficult to remove following post fracture or in the event of the need for endodontic retreatment.

Passive parallel sided serrated posts cemented with a non adhesive luting cement allows for easier post removal in the event of failure. Removal of metal posts is achieved by the application of an ultrasonic tip to the post under water coolant. This may be aided by removal of a limited amount of tooth tissue from around the post with a small round bur or a Masserann Kit (Fig 3-25a,b). The ultrasonic energy, transmitted to the post, breaks down the cement lute, allowing post removal.

Fig 3-25 (a,b) Fractured post seen in Fig 3-17 (a). To remove the post a trephine of slightly larger diameter than the post is chosen (Masserann) and used to create a "gutter" around the post. An ultrasonic tip is then used to shatter

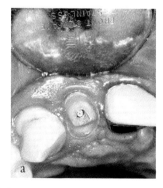
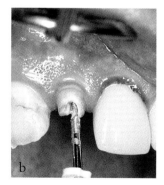

the cement lute and the trephine can again be used to remove the post (b). Removal of posts using this technique has a low risk of root fracture.

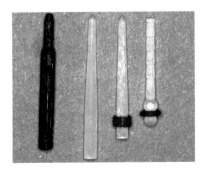

Fig 3-26 Fibre based posts: from left to right, carbon fibre post (Composipost, RTD, France) and three translucent quartz fibre posts (two smooth sided and one serrated), the DT Light-Post (RTD France), Luscent Anchor post (Dentatus, Sweden) and Para-Post Fiber Lux (Coltène Whaledent Ltd).

A relatively recent addition to the available range of preformed posts available is the fibre based post (Fig 3-26). Quartz fibre posts have glass fibres running longitudinally along the post length which are embedded in a composite material (Fig 3-27a,b). These posts are normally smooth sided as cutting serrations can weaken the fibre structure. Fibre posts are cemented into place with adhesive resin luting cement which bonds to the post and root dentine. Some root reinforcement may therefore be offered. The quartz fibre alignment also makes the posts strongly resistant to fracture, but allows some microscopic flexure similar to dentine under occlusal loads. In cases of post fracture or endodontic retreatment, fibre posts are removed by inserting a pin drill down the centre of the post, creating a pilot hole for the subsequent use of an instrument such as a Peezo reamer or small sized tapered post drill (Fig 3-28). When cut in alignment with the fibres, the post should be relatively easy to remove. Carbon fibre posts were introduced, but because they were black, they were superseded by white, tooth-coloured or clear quartz

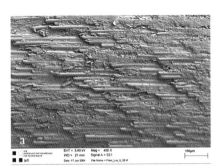
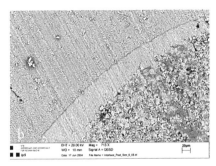

Fig 3-27 (a,b) Micrograph of the surface of a Fiber Lux quartz fibre post, showing the fibres running longitudinally along the post embedded in a composite material (a). Once cemented and cut in cross section, the micrograph shows the dentine (b), the intervening luting cement and the post (bottom right) (Courtesy of Coltène Whaledent Ltd).

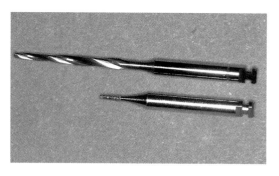

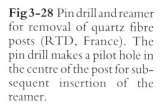

Fig 3-28 Pin drill and reamer for removal of quartz fibre posts (RTD, France). The pin drill makes a pilot hole in the centre of the post for subsequent insertion of the reamer.

fibre posts. Quartz fibre posts are ideal in combination with composite cores to support all-ceramic crowns. This results in a restoration that is completely tooth coloured and allows for optimum translucency and aesthetics.

Choice of Core Material

Selecting the correct core material for anterior or single rooted teeth should be relatively straightforward. Composite is the material of choice. When used in conjunction with an all-ceramic crown and resin luting cement, there is opportunity to create a totally bonded restored tooth unit. Some manufacturers produce a dual-cured fibre reinforced composite. This dual cured material is suitable for use in core formers and once the core former is removed the core can be modified accordingly (Fig 3-29).

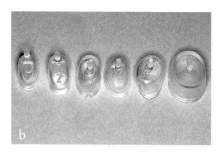

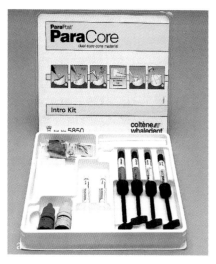

Fig 3-29 (a,b) Chemically cured fibre reinforced composite core material (a), also available in gun and double helix mixer tips (ParaCore, Coltène Whaledent Ltd), and clear core formers for different tooth type (b).

Appropriate core materials for posterior teeth include; amalgam, conventional and fibre reinforced composites. In situations where little coronal tooth tissue remains, amalgam cores tend to fracture on removal of the matrix band. This can be overcome by placing an orthodontic band around the tooth, packing the amalgam and leaving the band around the tooth until a second visit, when the amalgam has set. Alternatively, if orthodontic bands are not available a copper band can be trimmed and placed instead (Fig 3-30). However, the fit of these may not be as good as with an orthodontic band. Crown preparation may need to be deferred until any gingival inflammation induced by the plaque retentive band has subsided. To avoid this scenario, it is wise to leave the band in place for as short a time as possible.

Where good isolation is possible, consideration should be given to alternative materials such as composites. Composite cores can be shaped, prepared and an impression recorded in one visit. Even when root filled, a temporary crown is essential to prevent overeruption, mesial drift and tilting of adjacent teeth. There is a theoretical risk that if the composite core is not covered, swelling of the composite can occur in a moist environment, preventing the seating of the definitive crowns. This problem can be overcome by painting die relief on the master die prior to making of the crown.

It is important that a core material is sufficiently viscous and is readily packable within the preparation. Materials such as some conventional and resin-modified glass-ionomer cements are not viscous enough to pack and occasionally do not fully adapt to the cavity walls. When a final impression is taken the wash material will flow into the deficiencies, creating a fin in the final impression. This may not have a major impact on the final restoration, providing the majority of the core material is adapted and bonded to tooth tissue, and there is sufficient mechanical retention within the cavity. In this

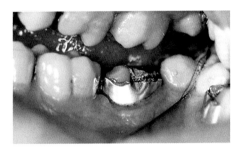

Fig 3-30 Copper band placed on a lower molar tooth to allow placement of an amalgam where little coronal tooth tissue remains. The amalgam is allowed to set and the band cut off a few days later. The band should not be left in place for extended periods as it has the potential to cause periodontal problems.

situation, however, it is essential that all preparation margins are on tooth tissue, as this will ensure the defect between core and remaining tooth tissue will fill with luting cement. As a general rule where tooth coloured restorative materials are concerned, preparation margins should be extended apically on to tooth tissue.

Further Reading

Ricketts DN, Tait CM, Higgins AJ. Tooth preparation for post-retained restorations. Br Dent J 2005;198:463-471.

Ricketts DN, Tait CM, Higgins AJ. Post and core systems, refinements to tooth preparation and cementation. Br Dent J 2005;198:533-541.

Sorensen JA, Martinoff JT. Intracoronal reinforcement and coronal coverage: a study of endodontically treated teeth. J Prosthet Dent 1984;51:780-784.

Sorensen JA, Martinoff JT. Endodontically treated teeth as abutments. J Prosthet Dent 1985;53:631-636.

Tait CM, Ricketts DN, Higgins AJ. Restoration of the root-filled tooth: pre-operative assessment. Br Dent J 2005;198:395-404.

Tait CM, Ricketts DN, Higgins AJ. Weakened anterior roots – intraradicular rehabilitation. Br Dent J 2005;198:609-617.

Chapter 4

Choosing the Right Crown

Aim

The aim of this chapter is to consider what factors are important when choosing the type of crown, and how to select the best materials to use.

Objective

After reading this chapter, the reader will be better able to judge which type of crown and what material should be used in a particular situation.

Introduction

There is an increasing range of crowns with a variety of physical properties. Crowns can, however, be conveniently classified into four main types:

- metal (usually gold alloys)
- metal–ceramic
- all–ceramic
- composite.

The clinician needs to weigh up the "pros" and "cons" of alternative crowns and advise the patient on the most suitable type for a given situation. This choice will be determined by general factors such as cost and preoperative factors, including the extent and type of existing restoration.

General Factors

Most patients want a tooth-coloured smile and would prefer not to show any metal restorations. Therefore, metal–ceramic and all–ceramic crowns are preferred for restoring teeth within the smile line. This has an impact upon cost and the amount of preparation required to successfully complete the crownwork. The results obtained with all–ceramic and metal–ceramic crowns can be excellent, but the end result is highly dependant upon the skill of the dental team. The clinician needs to complete a satisfactory preparation with sufficient horizontal and vertical space required to accommodate an aesthetically pleasing crown. In everyday practice the choice between different types of crown is often a question of the price the patient can afford to pay.

Preoperative Factors

Tooth Related Factors
Crowns are expensive; preoperative assessment of a tooth prior to considering a crown is therefore an important part of the decision making process. There are obvious assessments to make, such as vitality, periradicular status, quality of any root filling, inclination of the tooth and the occlusion. When deciding on the type of material for a crown, it is important to consider:
- the size of the restoration
- the core
- the position of the margin
- the vertical and horizontal space available
- the occlusal load
- the extent of tooth wear (Chapter 8)
- availability of appropriate technical support (Fig 4-1 and Fig 4-2).

The Size of Restoration
The performance and appearance of modern direct composite restorative materials is so good that there is no longer a pressing need to prepare extensively broken down teeth for crowns. The advantage of composite materials is that they can be repaired at the chair-side and maintained for long periods of time (Fig 4-3). The average survival for composites is 3–5 years and for crowns it is 10 years, but composites have the advantage of being more conservative of tooth tissue. Provided the repairs are not continuous and that there are reasonable time intervals of at least a year between appointments, composites can be maintained over many years. Once the

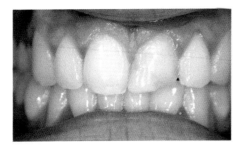

Fig 4-1 The fracture of the upper central incisor compromises the smile of this patient. The length and width of the restoration should mimic the adjacent teeth.

maintenance periods reduce to every 3–6 months, the time and cost of repairing composites becomes uneconomical.

The Margin

The optimal position for the gingival margin of a crown is on natural tooth just within the gingival sulcus (Fig 4-4). This hides the margin of the crown, limits plaque accumulation and offers the best opportunity of ideal marginal adaptation. This ideal situation can be difficult to achieve. Without an

Fig 4-2
The restorations placed on the patient seen in Fig 4-1. The margins of the crown are at the gingival margin, and in some areas just into the gingival crevice. If the patient maintains good oral hygiene, drift of the margin will be

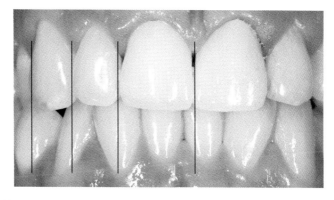

limited. The vertical lines highlight the concept of the golden proportion. The width of the central incisor is dominant and the relative widths of the lateral incisor and canine are incrementally narrower.

Fig 4-3 Composites have been placed along the incisal edges of these worn incisors and maintained for five years with annual refinishing. The appearance and translucency of modern composites provides aesthetically pleasing restorations which conserve tooth tissue.

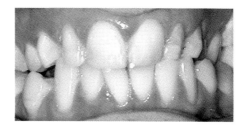

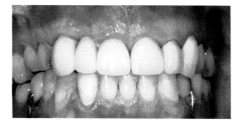

Fig 4-4 Margins of a crown at or around the gingival margin will remain more stable than those which are placed subgingivally.

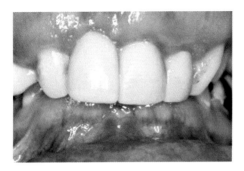

Fig 4-5 The margins on these anterior crowns have been placed subgingivally. The visible halo of the darkened gingival margin is apparent. If the patient is susceptible to periodontal disease the margin will continue to migrate apically eventually becoming exposed. This is a case in which crown lengthening should have preceded the provision of crowns.

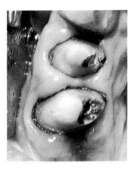

Fig 4-6 Teeth with subgingival margins are difficult to restore with crowns. Good soft tissue management can allow an acceptable impression to be taken. If the margins cannot be clearly recorded in an impression, either crown lengthening is indicated or a crown is contraindicated.

accurate impression of the margin, the longevity of the restoration will be compromised (Fig 4-5). A common dilemma is an extensively restored tooth needing a crown which has subgingival margins (Fig 4-6). A possible compromise is to finish the preparation for the crown on the core material and so provide a more favourable situation for the impression. Unfortunately, relying on two margins, one between the tooth and core and the other between the core and the crown, means an increased risk of early failure. In these circumstances, consideration should be given either to using an alternative to a crown, or to surgically repositioning the gingival margin apically to create a longer clinical crown.

The periodontal health of the gingiva surrounding a crown will, in part, be dependent upon the emergence profile of the crown. A good profile should mimic the contour of the tooth prior to the restoration. The preparation should remove sufficient tooth to allow the technician to develop a favourable crown profile. Overbuilding the crown creates an unfavourable emergence profile, increasing the risk of plaque accumulation and making cleaning more difficult. Under-preparing teeth, although conservative of tooth tissue, may have other consequences for gingival health (Fig 4-7a,b).

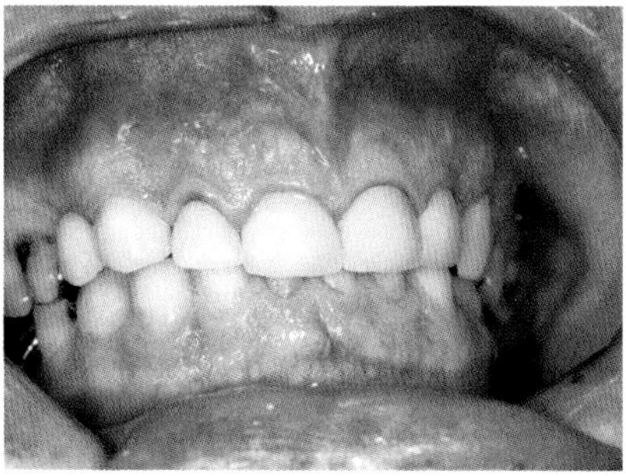

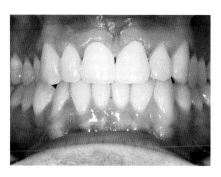

Fig 4-7a These anterior crowns have been overbuilt because insufficient tooth was removed. Such overbuilt crowns make maintenance of oral hygiene difficult.

Fig 4-7b The emergence profile of these crowns is in harmony with the adjacent teeth, giving a pleasing result. There is, however, a small black triangle between the two central incisors. Increasing the width of the teeth to hide the triangle would increase the contact area making the crown appear wider. The compromise of accepting a small black triangle was accepted.

The Core

Most teeth that are crowned will have an existing core restoration. The choice of a full or partial coverage crown, will have an impact upon the retention of the core. For example, crowns prepared on premolar and molar teeth with extensive amalgam MOD restorations present a particular problem.

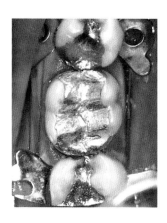

Fig 4-8 Removal of the buccal and lingual walls for a full coverage crown will result in loss of retention for the core. Preparation for a partial gold crown would retain walls which help retain and support the core.

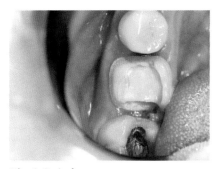

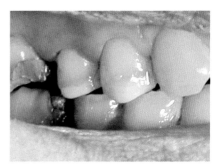

Fig 4-9 A three-quarter crown or cuspal coverage overlay conserves the lingual and buccal walls. The restoration can be made from porcelain, indirect composite or gold.

Fig 4-10 An extracoronal indirect composite has been used to restore the premolar teeth. Although the margins are visible, the design allowed the buccal wall to be retained to maintain the integrity of the core.

Amalgams are classically retained by undercuts on the buccal and lingual walls. Crown preparation may remove the support and retention of the core (Fig 4-8). An alternative crown design such as a three-quarter or cuspal coverage overlay can overcome these difficulties (Fig 4-9). Alternatively, an all-ceramic inlay or onlay directly luted to the tooth with an adhesive cement may conserve the buccal and lingual walls (Fig 4-10). The common dilemma is whether to provide a full or partial coverage crown on an extensively restored posterior tooth. A partial coverage overlay may be preferable to a full coverage metal-ceramic crown, but patient preference, vertical and horizontal space and clinical crown height are also important issues to consider.

The situation with anterior teeth is somewhat different. Here the need is to provide good aesthetics while maximising preservation of tooth tissue. While preserving tooth tissue is important, a visible junction between porcelain and tooth in partial coverage overlays typically results in an unacceptable outcome.

Vertical Space

The occlusal reduction needed for a metal-ceramic crown is greater than that for a metal onlay. The space needed for metal-ceramic occlusal coverage is around 1.5 mm. For all-ceramic crowns the space needed is nearer 1.5–2 mm. This is to provide sufficient space for an adequate thickness of ceramic, the material being relatively weak in thin section. Providing a metal occlusal surface can conserve tooth tissue and be useful when vertical space is compromised. However, in the mandible the metal will show, in particular, on first molars and premolars. Reducing occlusal surfaces to accommodate all-ceramic restorations cannot be considered a conservative procedure and is typically unsuitable for short clinical crowns.

Horizontal/Labial Space

The importance of horizontal/labial space is most apparent in metal-ceramic and all-ceramic crowns. Sufficient tooth needs to be removed to allow the technician to achieve acceptable aesthetics buccally. The ideal space is around 1.5 mm. This requires the removal of a substantial amount of tooth tissue. A graduated periodontal probe is useful in assessing the amount of tooth tissue removed (Fig 4-11). Alternatively, a preoperative silicone matrix can be taken of the tooth. After preparation, the matrix is replaced over the preparation and the amount of tooth tissue removed can be seen against the outline of the silicone impression (Fig 4-12).

The need for sufficient horizontal space is especially obvious for anterior crowns in patients with prominent anterior guidance, as seen in a Class II division II incisal relationship. The close proximity of the palatal surface of upper and the buccal surface of the lower incisors increases the difficulty of the preparation and control of the occlusion of crowns on these teeth. Careful palatal tooth reduction should be carried out to provide sufficient space for the crown, but it will be at a premium. The same problem presents in cases with high cuspal inclines and a lack of anterior guidance as seen in patients with a Class II division I or Class III incisal relationship (see Chapter 7).

Occlusal Load

The relevance of occlusal loading is especially important when considering an all-ceramic crown. If a patient has a history of bruxism or other para-

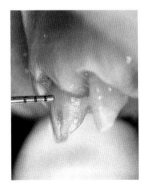 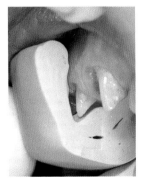

Fig 4-11 (left) Periodontal dental probe showing the amount of buccal reduction. The optimum amount of tooth reduction for a metal-ceramic crown is 1.5 mm.

Fig 4-12 (right) A matrix used to assess the optimum amount of tooth reduction.

functional activity, metal alloys are indicated for occlusal coverage. This is because ceramics may crack or fracture under repeated, high occlusal loads.

Technical Skill

One of the most important factors in the success of a crown is the skill of the technician in making the crown, in particular ceramic crowns. Many commercial laboratories produce crowns in stages with different technicians completing each stage. This may be cost-effective, but it may reduce the opportunity for liaison between the technician and the clinician. This liaison is very important in making crowns and inlays.

Selecting the Appropriate Crown

The choice between all-ceramic and metal-ceramic crowns is often determined by cost. Provided the patient can afford the more expensive all-ceramic crown and there is space for sufficient tooth preparation, the only contraindications to all-ceramic crowns are signs of bruxism (increased risk of fracture) and tooth wear (damage to the opposing unrestored teeth).

Posterior teeth can have indirect intra- or extracoronal restorations. Intracoronal restorations have the advantage of conserving tooth tissue. Although three-quarter crowns are not as common as they were, they still have a role in coronal coverage of root-filled teeth with extensive MOD restorations and minimal preparation bridgework (Fig 4-8). Where a full coverage crown preparation might result in the loss of the buccal or lingual cusp and hence retention for the core, a cuspal coverage overlay or three-quarter crown might preserve sufficient tooth tissue to retain the core (Fig 4-9). Gold has however, the disadvantage of unacceptable appearance to some patients, while all-ceramics need significant occlusal clearance. The choice of which material to use will vary between cases. Although gold is not always acceptable to patients a surprising number will accept it if the benefits of the material are explained to them. Indeed, for some this may be culturally or fashionably preferred. Above all else, it is important that the patient has a choice and is involved in the decision making process.

Materials

Metals

Metallic indirect restorations are generally made using the lost wax technique. This involves adapting a wax pattern to the working die, investing the pattern, burning out the wax under high temperature and replacing it

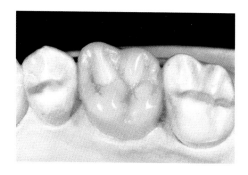

Fig 4-13 Wax pattern for a metal-ceramic crown (Courtesy of E Wnuk).

with molten metal which, on cooling, solidifies to the pattern left by the wax (Fig 4-13). Remembering that the technician needs to adapt wax to a die is important. If the clinician removes insufficient tooth when preparing the crown, the technician is left with insufficient space to rebuild the tooth in wax. A sufficient bulk of wax is needed to give the wax pattern sufficient strength to be removed from the stone die. A minimal preparation makes this impossible, without overbuilding the restoration.

Most metal alloys include gold to a greater or lesser extent. There are many classifications of gold alloys which are related to the gold content, but the one in common use is Type I to IV. Type I has a high gold content and it is used for inlays as the metal is quite malleable, Type IV is hard and normally used for gold partial denture bases. Types II and III are of increasing hardness and are used for crowns and bridges.

Base metals can be added to gold to create alloys of different physical properties. The choice is partly determined by economic needs, as the price of the base metals can vary. The noble alloys contain high gold content with small concentrations of platinum and palladium. The whiter the metal, the higher the concentration of noble metals, varying from 60–80% palladium. Non-precious alloys containing nickel or chromium result in a reduction in palladium and platinum, but as a consequence the accuracy of the casting is reduced. The metals used for metal-ceramic crowns need to have a high melting point as high firing temperatures are required for the addition of porcelain.

Ceramics

Conventional ceramics contain silicone dioxide and aluminium dioxide, with varying additions of others materials called fluxes (boron, potassium, sodium, magnesium, lithium oxides) – the resultant mix is commonly referred to as feldspathic porcelain. Aluminous porcelain is strengthened by crystalline alumina. This increases tensile and flexural strength and may hinder crack propagation. The addition of leucite to porcelain increases the resistance to fracture as does zirconia which stops crack growth.

For metal-ceramic crowns, the porcelain is added in layers. The inner opaque porcelains are added to mask the metal and over this aesthetic porcelains are added to produce the shape and shade of the crown. Although the cores used for all-ceramic crowns are not made of metal, they are quite often opaque and need masking. This means that the bright and opaque porcelain coping, like that of metal, needs masking to create optimum aesthetics. A reduction in the use of metal-ceramic restorations is popular with dentists and the public.

All-ceramic materials can be classified as follows:
- CAD/CAM
- Castable – pressed
- Conventional.

CAD/CAM

In some computer-aided-design/computer-aided-manufacture (CAD/CAM) crown systems the coping is produced by a computer driven scanner which digitises the working die in the laboratory and sends data to a centralised laboratory in either the USA or Sweden (Fig 4-14). The coping is then manufactured by a computer controlled milling process to produce a thimble shaped coping of high strength which is returned to the original laboratory. Conventional porcelains are laid on the coping to shape and colour the crown (Fig 4-15a,b). The advantage of the computer controlled milling process is a crown with a very high precision fit, in particular along the margins. The coping can either be 0.4 or 0.6 mm thick. This can influence the amount of tooth removed to provide space for the crown. The thinner coping, which is not as strong as

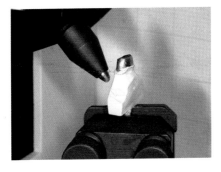

Fig 4-14 The Procera machine uses a ruby sapphire probe to scan the master die. The data collected is digitally stored and e-mailed to a centralised laboratory. The core is returned to the local technician to complete the crown.

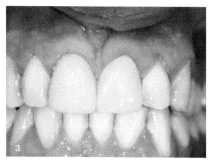 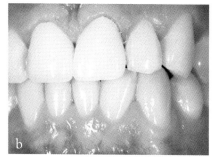

Fig 4-15 (a,b) Procera all-ceramic crowns (b) have been used to replace unacceptable metal-ceramic crowns (a).

the thick coping, allows the first to be used in areas where space is limited and further tooth reduction is not possible. This might be for example in occlusal contact areas on teeth with short clinical crowns.

CAD/CAM without coping, e.g. Cerec III (Sirona, Germany)

Unlike, the Procera system, the Cerec III system optically captures an image intraorally and then transmits the data to computer controlled milling machines. The system produces a crown, inlay or coping. Like castable ceramics the colour of the crown or inlay is typically homogenous, but there are some blocks of ceramic with different layers of chroma. The system mills blocks of ceramic into the crown or inlays within 10–20 minutes, with an accuracy of fit similar to that of other milled crowns. The finished crown or inlay can be characterised by a technician by adding porcelains to the surface of the milled crown. Milled copings are layered with conventional porcelains to form crowns.

Castable

Like Procera, this type of crown (e.g. Empress I/II (Ivoclar Vivadent)) comprises two layers. The bulk of the crown is made from an ingot of Empress I/Empress II. Once cast, using the lost wax technique, surface features may be added by using conventional low fusing porcelains (Fig 4-16a,b).

Conventional

This type of crown (e.g. Inceram (Vita Zahnfabrik)) consists of two distinct layers. As in a Procera crown strength comes from the inner core. Surface features are added by removing thin sections of Inceram and replacing them

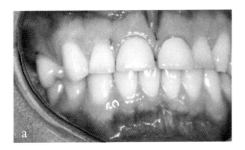

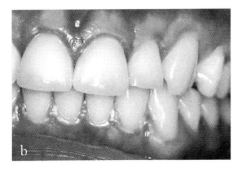

Fig 4-16 (a,b) Empress crowns are made by the lost wax technique and then cut back to characterise the buccal surfaces. The original metal-ceramic crowns were dull and lifeless. The replacement crowns appear natural and vital.

with conventional porcelains. Again, in a similar manner to Procera, the appearance can be compromised by the core, which is strong but opaque (Fig 4-17). Conventional low fusing porcelains are applied over the core to create an aesthetically pleasing high strength crown.

Shell Crowns (Resin Bonded/Dentine Bonded Crowns)

The term shell crown is used to describe a thin conventional porcelain crown bonded to the tooth. These crowns are thinner than conventional porcelain crowns. Strength is derived from the bond between the luting cement and the tooth or core substrate. The resin interface resists crack propagation, pro-

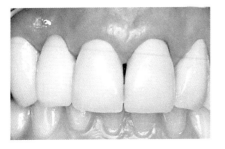

Fig 4-17 Inceram crowns have been used to restore these anterior teeth. Like Procera and Empress crowns, Inceram crowns require some cut back to create space for individual characterisation of the labial surface. This is achieved with conventional porcelains. The crowns could have been widened to hide the interproximal areas without compromising the appearance of the crowns.

viding sufficient strength within the crown for the restoration of most anterior teeth and, in some circumstances, posterior teeth.

Clinical Indications

Although modern all-ceramic crowns are stronger than conventional porcelain crowns, long-term performance remains to be determined. There are some concerns over the clinical performance of these restorations compared with metal-ceramic crowns, but they offer metal free alternatives which continue to undergo rapid technical development. Most laboratories will, for economic reasons, provide only one type of all-ceramic crown. Choice may therefore be limited unless a different laboratory is chosen. In any of the layering techniques, as in metal-ceramic crownwork (Fig 4-18) the outcome is dependant upon the skill of the technician. There may be some justification to use porcelain shell type crowns rather than all-ceramic crowns in situations where occlusal loading is reduced, for example on lower incisors.

Colour Matching

Different porcelain manufacturers produce slightly different porcelains. Also different batches of porcelain from the same manufacturer will have slight variations even within the same shade. Therefore, if multiple crowns are being placed there is the temptation to make the crowns at the same time but care must be taken to control the occlusion, contact points and anterior guidance. In some circumstances abnormalities in the tooth form can be matched on the crowns (Fig 4-19). Otherwise, there may be subtle differences in colour, ren-

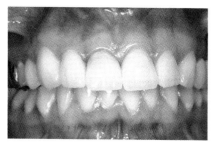 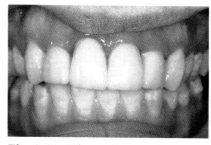

Fig 4-18 Metal-ceramic crowns used in the appropriate circumstance can have an acceptable appearance, even in demanding situations with the advantages of strength and endurance.

Fig 4-19 These all-ceramic crowns have been made to mimic fluoritic stains present in the adjacent natural teeth.

dering the restorations unacceptable. The most difficult clinical situation is to match a single crown to otherwise unrestored anterior teeth (Fig 4-1).

Shade Taking

The ideal time to take a shade is at the beginning of treatment before the teeth become dehydrated and lighter. Most patients' teeth lie within similar colour ranges. For instance using the Vita Classic Guide (Vitapan Classical) young patients' teeth are normally A2, older patients' teeth are A3 or A3.5. If the colour of a tooth is judged to be in the C or D shades, then it is worthwhile reassessing the shade to ensure that the colour match is correct. Various manufacturers are attempting to link laboratory processing of the crowns with digital photography and photospectroscopy in the dental surgery. In time, this process may become more reliable, but at the present most shades are recorded manually at the chair-side in good lighting or under daylight corrected lights.

Tooth Shape

The shape of the crown can be conveniently described in terms of:
• length and width
• position of the gingival margin
• incisal edge
• relationship to the upper and lower lips
• contact areas.

Length and Width

Ideally, for anterior teeth a crown should be longer than it is wide; the ratio should be around 1:0.75 to 1:0.8. Crowns which are made too long appear unnatural (Fig 4-5). Crowns with a balanced length to width ratio appear more natural and are aesthetically pleasing (Fig 4-15). When the width to length ratio increases, the tooth appears square and unnatural.

The illusion of perspective is also important for the appearance of teeth. As objects appear further distant, they appear narrower. The relationship between the width of upper central, lateral incisors and canines remains relatively constant. The central incisors being the most anterior teeth appear prominent when looked at from in front. The lateral incisors appear slightly less wide and, correspondingly, the canines appear narrower than the laterals and so on. The teeth appear narrower the further back they are located in the mouth. This relationship is considered to follow the golden proportion (Fig 4-2).

Position of the Gingival Margin

The position of the gingival margin is important to the aesthetic appearance of a crown. Although it is not always possible to achieve, the upper lateral incisor's gingival margin should be slightly coronal to that of the central incisor and canine (Fig 4-2). When the gingival margins lie at the same level, the appearance can be less attractive (Fig 4-3). If the crown's margins are uneven, the appearance, although acceptable, is not necessarily the most pleasing (Fig 4-4). Control of the gingival contour is important and this is described in Chapter 6. No matter how carefully teeth are prepared, there is a likelihood that the margin between the tooth and the crown will eventually show. If gingival margins and, in turn, margins of crowns are included in the smile, consideration should be given to alternative restorative options prior to embarking on the crown work.

Incisal Edge

The incisal position of the teeth can be critical to their appearance. The central incisors should be slightly longer than the lateral incisors, but the same length as the canines (Fig 4-2). When the teeth are worn the incisal height becomes even (Fig 4-3). Uneven incisal edges (Fig 4-16a,b) while not unappealing, are not as pleasing as a stepped appearance (Fig 4-4). Although the incisal position of the crowns in Fig 4-4 approaches the acceptable, the position of the gingival margin and the length to width ratio make these restorations look like crowns rather than teeth.

Lips

The position of the upper and lower lips in relation to a crown can influence the acceptability of the appearance of the restoration. In some cases, the incisal relationship between the upper and lower anterior teeth may compromise appearance. Class II division I and II situations create teeth with proclined or retroclined incisors respectively. The lips hide the teeth in a Class II division II case. In a Class II division I relationship the teeth are exposed. Without orthodontic treatment, the appearance is unlikely to be improved by restorative management alone. In patients with a Class I incisal relationship, about one third of the crown should show when smiling.

The curve of the upper and lower lips is important to having a "nice smile". Ideally, the curve of the lower lips and the upper anterior teeth should match. Opposite curves provide an unpleasing appearance.

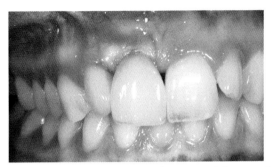

Fig 4-20 The incisal edge of the crown on the upper right central incisor is more translucent in this young patient. The translucency is mimicked by using porcelains with a blue tint. The mismatch of the width of the central incisors has to some extent been hidden by increasing the width of the crown on the upper right central incisor. A consequence of this increased width is the black triangle. Elimination of this triangle would be difficult to achieve.

Contact Areas

Ideally, the contact between adjacent anterior teeth should be placed towards the incisal third of the tooth and cover a few millimetres. A long contact area will tend to emphasise a square shaped tooth and may reflect the appearance of a worn tooth. The contact area between teeth in younger patients tends to be positioned towards the incisal edge. The mesial incisal edge tends to be more angular than the distal, which is more curved.

A relatively common problem is the management of spaces between teeth. Diastemas occur frequently. In some cases minor increases in the width of the teeth can eliminate gaps. There is a limit, however, to how wide a tooth can be without compromising the aesthetic outcome. Once the ratio of the length to width of a tooth increases above 1:0.8 it appears too square. It may be possible to compensate for minor increases in width by increasing the length of a crown, within the limits of the occlusion. Also increases in width can be disguised to some extent by creating a more acute angle along the proximal contact areas of the crown, but the flexibility of this approach is limited (Fig 4-20). In general, any proposed increase in the width of a tooth should be trialled with a diagnostic wax-up. Alternatively, uncured composite can be added to the tooth to visualise the appearance of any changes.

Surface Finish of Crowns

Most natural teeth are not a homogenous colour. They are composed of various colours, reflecting the differing proportions of enamel and dentine present within the tooth. For example, the incisal edge of teeth, particularly in young patients, can appear translucent (Fig 4-20). This appearance is the result of an absence of dentine in the mesial and distal thirds of the incisal edge. The construction of the crown should mimic this appearance. From a clinical perspective, sufficient tooth reduction is needed to create space for the technician to achieve this outcome. The technician needs to add different coloured porcelains, often shades of blue, to the mesial and distal thirds of incisal edges to mimic natural translucency (Fig 4-20). Along the gingival margin the colour of the dentine is more prominent as the enamel is thin in this region – the colour tends to be more orange than yellow. This is particularly important in patients with some degree of gingival recession. In both situations the technician needs to be informed of these subtleties in the variation of colour in the crown.

Highly polished or glazed surfaces will reflect more light than rough surfaces which tend to scatter light. Relatively thick enamel in younger patients tends to be more reflective than thinned enamel in older patients. Furthermore, as teeth age and the enamel gradually reduces in thickness the colour of the underlying dentines becomes more dominant. A highly polished crown will look unnatural, and therefore the labial surface of the crown should be broken up with vertical zones replicating the mammelons of the natural tooth. Such factors enhance the appearance of teeth and crowns but are by no means critical. For most patients, achieving an acceptable aesthetic outcome is the priority. This, however, should not lessen the dentist's responsibility to optimise the clinical outcome – always strive for excellence.

Further Reading

Bartlett D, Fisher N. Clinical problem solving in prosthodontics. Edinburgh: Churchill Livingstone, 2003.

Smith BGN. Planning and making crowns and bridges. London: Martin Dunitz, 1998.

Chapter 5

Tooth Preparation

Aim

The aim of this chapter is to describe the common tooth preparations for crowns and how to achieve the best results.

Objective

After this chapter the reader will understand how to prepare teeth for crowns.

Cemented Crowns

Preparing teeth for crowns typically involves removing substantial quantities of enamel and dentine and as a consequence it is not a conservative technique. The aim of the preparation, in addition to creating space to accommodate the intended crown, is to prepare a shape appropriate to retain and support the crown. The ideal taper should be 10–20°. This is recognised to be sufficiently parallel to be retentive, yet tapered enough to remove a wax pattern from the stone model and allow cementation of the final crown (Fig 5-1a,b). A parallel-sided preparation mesiodistally increases the risk of either damage to the adjacent teeth, even when a fine tapered bur is used, or over-preparation of the tooth. Short preparations normally provide insufficient retention for conventionally luted crowns. Conversely, it is difficult to avoid creating undercuts in long preparations.

Preparations may cause death of the pulp – one of the most common complications following tooth reduction. The impact of preparation can be reduced by using copious water spray to dissipate the heat, but even then some pulps die as a result of the effects of excess heat on vital tissues. This most commonly occurs in teeth which are already compromised. Elective root treatment results in even more tooth tissue reduction and tends to limit the longevity of the tooth. A balance needs to be achieved between methods used to maintain pulpal vitality and the implications of having to root treat a tooth soon after crowning.

For most teeth, the amount of tooth tissue that needs to be removed should be sufficient to provide adequate space for the restoration whilst leaving as

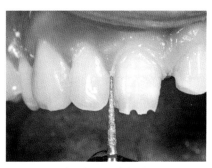

Fig 5-1a The shape of the bur can assist the preparation of an anterior tooth.

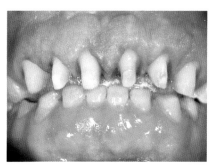

Fig 5-1b The taper of these preparations approaches parallel maximising the retention for the crowns.

much tooth tissue as possible to support the restoration and avoid damaging the pulp–dentine complex. Cutting should be intermittent and undertaken with copious water spray.

Burs

The shape of burs can help to achieve the appropriate shape and limit the amount of tooth reduction. Long thin tapered diamonds are ideal for proximal reduction. The taper is designed to create the optimum shape for retention and resistance form. Thicker burs are useful for occlusal, buccal and aspects of lingual reduction. For the reduction of the palatal surfaces of upper incisor teeth a rugby (oval) ball shaped bur creates the optimum shape to the tooth preparation (Fig 5-2).

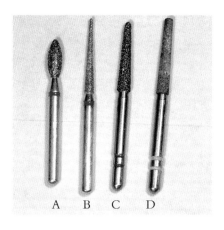

A   B   C   D

Fig 5-2 The bur shown in A is designed for preparation of the palatal surfaces of upper anterior teeth and the occlusal surfaces of molars. Bur B is useful for the margins of gold restorations. It has a fine taper for the proximal reduction of teeth. The end of the bur shown in C is too curved for a shoulder preparation for metal-ceramic crowns. A bur like D with a flat end would be more appropriate.

Requirements

- **Open proximal contact areas**
  The reason for open proximal contact areas (Fig 5-3) is found in the laboratory production of a crown. One of the first stages in making a crown is to section the model by sawing between prepared and adjacent teeth. It allows the technician access to trim the die. Failure to remove proximal contacts would leave the technician needing to saw through part of the preparation in an attempt to separate the model. This would result in an inaccurate die and consequently an ill-fitting crown.

- **Space for the restoration**
  Different types of restoration need differing amounts of space. A metal-ceramic crown needs sufficient tooth reduction to make space for the metal and porcelain. All-ceramic crowns need even more space, in particular, occlusally because the porcelain is weak in thin section. Gold crowns need the least amount of tooth reduction because of their strength.

- **Rounded angles**
  When the preparation is complete the clinician should remove sharp angles, otherwise, when the impression is cast, the sharp angles can be easily abraded or chipped in the laboratory production. If a crown is made to a damaged die it may not fully seat on the tooth (Fig 5-4).

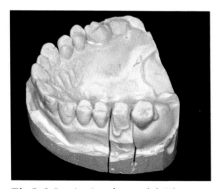

Fig 5-3 Sectioning the model. The contact areas between the teeth should be cleared otherwise sectioning cuts will pass through the preparation.

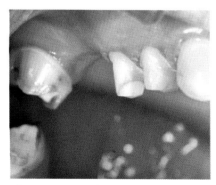

Fig 5-4 Leaving sharp line angles can lead to problems with the seating of crowns. The working model will have sharp edges which may wear. If this occurs, the crown may not seat accurately, leaving a gap at the gingival margin.

73

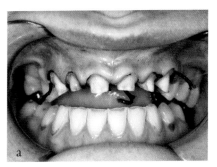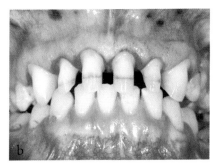

Fig 5-5 (a,b) The preparations in (a) have short clinical crowns which lack retention and resistant form. This is in contrast to the preparations seen in (b).

- *Retention and resistance form*
  For most conventional crowns, the shape of the preparation will determine the retention of the crown (Fig 5-5a,b). There are some minor differences in tooth preparation between the various types of crown and inlay preparations.

Extracoronal Restorations

There are two main methods of preparing the tooth – freehand which often results in overpreparation, or using depth slots and grooves to ensure optimum tooth reduction. Depth grooves may appear to some to be unnecessary, but are especially useful in avoiding overpreparation. They should follow the original contour of the tooth so that the crown becomes a veneer of uniform thickness. This element of the preparation is readily achieved using a long parallel sided bur (Fig 5-1).

Stages in Crown Preparation

Occlusal/Incisal Reduction

Assess the position, shape and orientation of the unprepared tooth. This might be best achieved with the aid of a preoperative study cast. An overerupted or inclined opposing tooth may require adjustment to correct the occlusal plane. Following occlusal modification, the tooth being crowned may require limited occlusal reduction as sufficient interocclusal space may have been achieved with the adjustment of the opposing tooth (Fig 5-6). In most cases, 1.5 mm clearance is needed, unless a metal occlusal surface is planned.

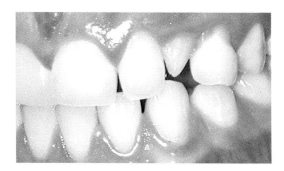

Fig 5-6 Occlusal reduction is not needed for the upper left peg lateral incisor as there is already sufficient interocclusal space.

Buccal/Lingual Reduction

It is largely personal preference as to whether the proximal or buccal/lingual reduction is done first (Fig 5-7). The buccal surface of a tooth has a complex shape and is often divided into the gingival, mid-buccal and occlusal/incisal contours (Fig 5-8a,b). The occlusal or incisal contour is one of the most important features of a crown preparation as it directly influences the shape of the crown. Too little tooth reduction means that insufficient space is created for the crown and leads to an overbuilt crown. If there is not enough space the technician needs to reduce the amount of porcelain covering the metal or ceramic coping which leads to a restoration which is too bright, as the underlying core shows through. Alternatively, the crown is over contoured to mask the coping, but this results in a compromised clinical outcome (Fig 5-9). This is a particular problem cervically as overcontouring creates an inappropriate emergence profile, plaque accumulation and periodontal problems. Limited lingual reduction is needed for a metal-ceramic crown as there is no need for porcelain on this surface.

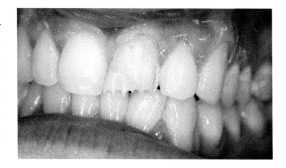

Fig 5-7 Grooves can be placed to control the depth of the buccal reduction. The depth cut shown is sufficient to provide space for a metal-ceramic crown. If the depth cut is started about 1 mm above the planned position for the gingival margin there is greater control over the preparation.

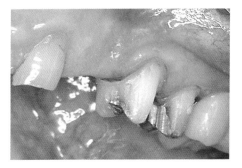

Fig 5-8a The buccal reduction should include a gingival, mid-buccal and an incisal reduction to match the contour of the tooth. If insufficient tooth is removed buccally, the technician either overbuilds the crown, or maintains the contour but produces an opaque restoration, as there is insufficient porcelain to mask the underlying metal.

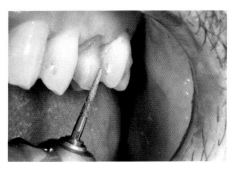

Fig 5-8b Following the contour of the tooth produces the optimum space for the crown.

Proximal Surfaces

Proximal surfaces are possibly the most demanding aspect of preparations. Most preparations involve, to a greater or lesser extent, some damage to the adjacent teeth. It is possible to reduce the damage by using long thin tapered burs or protecting the adjacent teeth with, for example, a matrix. The bur should be placed just within the bulk of the tooth so that it passes through the proximal area. The aim should be to leave a thin slither of tooth or core between the bur and adjacent tooth (Fig 5-1a). Once through the contact area the thin slither of tooth can be broken off and the margin smoothed. Despite this precaution damage to the adjacent tooth or restoration is very common and it is important that it is identified and treated appropriately. For minimal damage which is often unseen, no intervention is needed. Marked damage, such as visible preparation lines on the adjacent enamel should be polished and treated with a fluoride application. More serious damage involving dentine is unacceptable but if it occurs the tissue should be protected with a resin-based material. Damage to adjacent restorations is often left untreated. This results in an increase in the area of contact between the teeth, increasing the risk of food packing and periodontal problems.

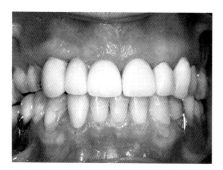

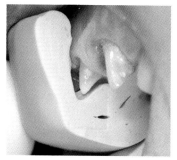

Fig 5-9 The upper right canine has been underprepared on its buccal surface. This has resulted in an overcontoured crown which does not conform to the outline of the arch.

Fig 5-10 The amount of buccal reduction can be checked with a matrix. The matrix is taken before preparation and then reinserted once the preparation is considered complete.

It is helpful to obtain a matrix impression before preparing a tooth to assist in assessing if adequate tooth reduction has been accomplished. The matrix should be sectioned buccolingually along the mid point of the tooth to be prepared. The matrix can be reinserted into the mouth to assess the depth of tooth reduction (Fig 5-10). Another method is to take an alginate impression and cast it in a fast setting plaster and to assess the preparation in the model. Using these methods it is possible to make critical adjustments to otherwise completed preparations.

Differences between Crowns

Metal–ceramic Crown

The ideal margins for a metal-ceramic crown are a shoulder buccally and a chamfer lingually. The shoulder is a 90° butt joint used to maximise the strength of the porcelain (Fig 5-11). Some clinicians prefer to have an additional chamfer for the metal, but most do not. The butt joint allows the technician to achieve a good quality, aesthetically pleasing gingival colour in the crown. Most butt ended burs have flat ends to create the desirable shoulder configuration. These burs can however, be quite narrow which may lead to peaks of tooth tissue along the gingival margin (Fig 5-12). Such peaks must be removed, otherwise they may be broken on the model, leading to a deficiency in the crown margin at fit. Alternatively, they may be lost at the time of cementation or early in clinical service, leaving a gap between the crown and the tooth. The margin should

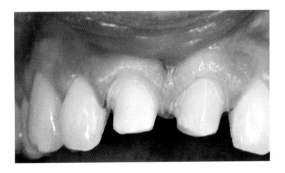

Fig 5-11 A butt joint is needed for metal-ceramic crowns to protect the porcelain which is brittle in thin section.

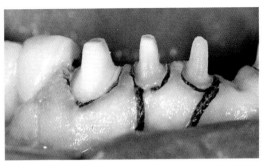

Fig 5-12 If ledges remain along the gingival margin, they will be replicated in the impression and cast. The sharp edges may be worn or chipped off the cast resulting in difficulties seating the completed crown.

follow the gingival contour around the tooth, avoiding trauma to the interdental papilla.

All-ceramic Crowns

More tooth reduction is needed for all-ceramic crowns than metal based ones. But the basic shape and procedure remains the same as for a metal-ceramic crown. On the occlusal, palatal or lingual surfaces at least 1.5 mm and preferably 2 mm of tooth reduction is needed. Some all-ceramic crowns are made using laser or contacting profilometers and these instruments do not record sharp line angles. It is important to ensure that the incisal edges are smoothed, and the margins prepared as 90° butt joints (Fig 5-13).

Three-quarter Crown

These crowns allow the buccal wall of the tooth to be preserved and are normally made in gold. This type of crown remains an ideal restoration for root-filled molar and premolar teeth. The occlusal, lingual and proximal tooth reduction is the same as for other preparations, but the buccal reduction differs in that only the occlusal 1–3 mm is prepared. Grooves should be cut along the long axis of the tooth on the mesial and distal surfaces as far buc-

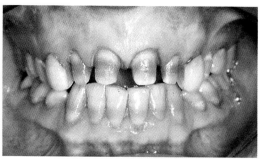

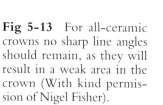

Fig 5-13 For all-ceramic crowns no sharp line angles should remain, as they will result in a weak area in the crown (With kind permission of Nigel Fisher).

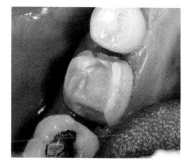

Fig 5-14 A three-quarter crown on a molar. It is difficult to avoid undercuts in such preparations.

cal as possible (Fig 5-14). These grooves increase retention of the crown. An offset occlusal groove joining the mesial and distal grooves can be used to create an arch of thickened gold, which resists distortion. In certain situations mesial and/or distal boxes can be substituted for grooves. This is especially useful if the three-quarter crown is used as a minor retainer for a fixed-moveable bridge. The metal margin is best finished as a chamfer. Despite some advantages three-quarter crowns are not commonly prescribed in practice. This is related to the demands of the preparation and most patients' dislike of displaying gold in their smile.

Cuspal Coverage Overlay
Cuspal overlay restorations are especially useful in protecting teeth with weakened buccal and lingual cusps – for example, teeth with extensive MOD restorations or subsequent to having been root filled. Like three-quarter crowns, the occlusal and proximal reduction is the same as for other types of crowns. The lingual and buccal reductions are, however, like the buccal reduction for three-quarter crowns. A classic MOD inlay preparation may be cut intracoronally. In such cases most of the retention for the restoration is obtained from the proximal boxes. The overlay needs to be designed to

79

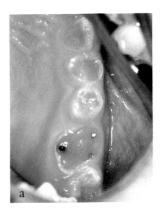
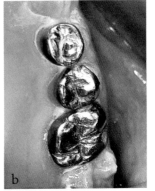

Fig 5-15 (a,b) These broken down teeth can be restored by means of composites. In similar cases crowns may be bonded directly to the remaining tooth tissue.

optimise the retention. The internal and external walls should be near parallel without creating undercuts. Like the three-quarter crown, most patients prefer not to have gold showing in the mouth. Cuspal coverage onlays can be made in ceramic and are popular with patients, but more occlusal reduction is needed for the porcelain.

Intracoronal Restorations

Metal Inlays

There are few indications for metal inlays in modern dental practice. This is partly a response to changing materials and a preference by many patients to have tooth-coloured restorations. Metal onlays still have a role, but less than they did. For this reason they are not now often prescribed (Fig 5-15a,b).

Porcelain Inlays

Adhesively cemented porcelain or composite inlays rely primarily on the cement lute for retention, which has some influence on the preparation. The essential requirements of an inlay are the same as for extracoronal restorations (Fig 5-16a,b). The inlay must be at least 1.5 mm thick to resist fracture. The depth and taper of the preparation aids retention and the support of the restoration. The preparations are, however, demanding; the number of internal lines makes it difficult to avoid undercuts. One manufacturer uses computer controlled milling, which is possible at the chair-side (Cerec III).

Indirect Composite Inlays

The qualities of indirect composite inlays are generally inferior to those of porcelain inlays. Although the composite is similar to that used at the chair-

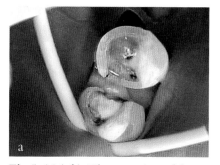
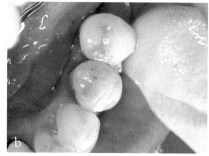

Fig 5-16 (a,b) The retention of the cuspal coverage all-ceramic onlay on the second premolar and the inlay on the first premolar will depend on the sufficiency of the adhesive composite lute.

side it is stronger and has greater wear resistance. As with porcelain inlays, if the surfaces are prepared near parallel, it may be difficult to remove the inlay from the die. A generous taper is needed to assist the technician. The adhesive provides most of the retention for the restoration.

Methods to Increase Retention

Slots and Grooves

Increasing the surface area of the preparation will increase the retention and resistance form of the restoration. Provided slots and grooves are prepared along the same paths of withdrawal as the external walls of the preparation, they will help to retain the restoration (Fig 5-17). If a slot or groove is too shallow, it may be filled with die relief material and, as a consequence, not included in the completed restoration. If a preparation is short or very tapered mesiodistally, grooves should be placed along the buccal and lingual walls. If the preparation is tapered buccolingually, then grooves should be placed mesially and distally.

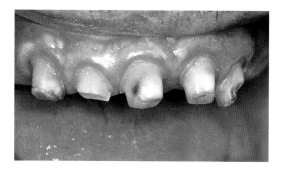

Fig 5-17 These grooves have been placed to increase mechanical retention by increasing the surface area of the preparation.

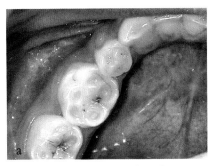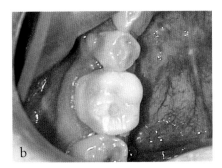

Fig 5-18 (a,b) A worn tooth surface. Some preparation should be undertaken to increase the surface area for bonding and to provide positive location for the restoration.

Resin-retained Indirect Restorations

Dentine bonding agents and adhesive luting cements have made resin-retained restorations reliable. For composite and porcelain inlays near parallel surfaces in the preparation increase the difficulty of making the restoration. As retention is derived from the cement lute, the overall objective of the preparation becomes the conservation and replacement of lost tooth tissue with composite or ceramic. The main difficulty in making these types of indirect restorations is the laboratory stage, since the restorations can be difficult to remove and reseat on the working cast.

A common indication for adhesively retained restorations is worn occlusal surfaces. The exposed dentine and enamel facilitates bonding, as little or no tooth reduction is needed, provided sufficient interocclusal space exists (Fig 5-18a,b and Fig 5-19). Another common indication for adhesive crowns is

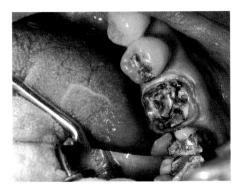

Fig 5-19 With virtually no coronal tooth tissue remaining, this tooth would have required either a pinned retained core and crown or elective root treatment and a post and core to retain a crown. An adhesively retained metal, porcelain or composite onlay, could restore the shape and function of the tooth without having to resort to conventional methods for retention.

replacement restorations. If removal of caries or an existing core leaves insufficient coronal tissue for conventional retention, the use of an adhesive cement should be considered as an alternative to elective root canal treatment and provision of a post crown.

Summary

Stages of Preparation
- Complete preoperative assessments, including radiographs, vitality tests and study models with diagnostic wax-up if necessary.
- Design the restoration.
- Administer local anaesthesia, as indicated clinically.
- Take putty matrix impression for provisional restoration.
- Take an additional matrix to check depth of preparation.
- Cut slots or grooves as a guide to depth reduction.
- Complete the buccal reduction, with gingival, mid-buccal and incisal reductions for extracoronal restorations.
- Prepare buccal shoulder, as appropriate for metal-ceramic restorations, or follow the same depth reduction all the way around the tooth for an all-ceramic crown.
- Prepare mesially and distally.
- Join the surfaces together to give a smooth even reduction.
- Remove sharp line angles.
- Check clearance.

Further Reading

Blair FM, Wassell RW, Steele JG. Crowns and other extra-coronal restorations: preparations for full veneer crowns. Br Dent J 2002;192:561-564,567-571.

Potts RG, Shillingburg HT Jr, Duncanson MG Jr. Retention and resistance of preparations for cast restorations. J Prosthet Dent 2004;92:207-212.

Chapter 6

Shade Taking, Provisional Crowns, Impressions and Cementation

Aim

The aim of this chapter is to describe how to take a shade, make provisional restorations, record impressions and to explain the value of taking interocclusal records.

Objective

After this chapter the reader will understand the importance of these critical stages in making crowns.

Introduction

Shade taking can be one of the more demanding aspects of providing crowns. Optimum results may be achieved by involving the technician in this important process. The role of the provisional restoration, in addition to covering, protecting and maintaining the position of the prepared tooth between appointments, is to assess the design, shape and occlusal relationship of the planned restoration. The term "temporary" infers that the life span of the restoration is short, but this may not be the case in complicated treatments. Therefore, the preferred term is provisional. The recording of impressions is a critical stage in making crowns as the information is used by the technician to make the restoration. Inadequate impressions are of no value and result in poor clinical results. Collaboration between dentist and technician is critical to clinical success. Cementation is the final stage in making crowns. Choosing the right cement is important in securing a long-lasting restoration. The luting process should never be rushed; it requires careful attention to detail.

Shade Taking

Following tooth assessment and diagnostic tests the first stage in the provision for a crown should be shade taking. This critical stage is commonly left to last by which time the tooth and adjacent teeth have dehydrated and become lighter. Ideally, the shade should be taken at the outset to reduce the risk of error.

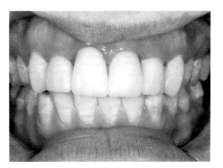 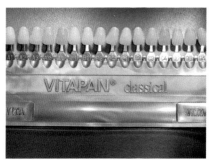

Fig 6-1 The laboratory sheet should include instructions to the technician on the shape, colour and the presence of features including translucency, speckles and surface characteristics.

Fig 6-2 Vita Classic shade guide.

The first requirement is to use natural light to take the shade. When this is not possible, a variety of shade taking lights may be used. If natural light is available, the patient should be taken to the window to record the shade. Using either technique, take short quick looks at the tooth rather than long stares. Longer views of the tooth bleach the retina and reduce the reliability of shade taking. Using a mirror, get agreement from the patient and record the agreed shade in the notes and on the prescription card. If individual characteristics such as speckles, incisal translucency, gingival staining are present, indicate these on the record (Fig 6-1).

If possible, provide a photograph or digital image of the tooth for the technician. Be careful in the use of incisal translucency, which tends to be present in young people. Incisal translucency in the older patient can appear unnatural.

A variety of shade guides are available. The most commonly used is the Vita Classic (Fig 6-2). This guide comprises A, B, C and D shade tabs, reflecting different hues. Each group is subdivided into chroma (saturation of colour). When using the guide the most common shades are A2 (younger patients), A3 (middle-aged patients) and A3.5 (older patients). Whilst this is not prescriptive, it is worth rechecking the shade if the chosen shade is markedly different. Other guides are arranged according to value (blackness/whiteness) and subdivided according to hue. Whichever shade guide is used, it is important to ensure that it is compatible with the materials used by the technician.

Provisional Crown

The use of acrylic crowns, made directly at the chair-side, has been superseded by resin composite crowns which are stronger and more likely to survive in the mouth. A role remains for acrylic provisional restorations, but this continues to diminish with time. The durability of acrylic provisional crowns can be improved if they are made in the laboratory. The advantage of long-term laboratory made acrylic crowns is that they are more resistant to stains, better contoured and accurately fit the preparation (Fig 6-3). Chair-side resin composite crowns offer similar advantages without laboratory costs.

A common mistake is to make the provisional restoration after taking the impression. The advantage of making the provisional restoration before taking the impression is that the preparation can be assessed for adequate reduction and undercuts. It is also useful for time management, in particular if the impression stage is prolonged. With the provisional restoration made, the appointment can be quickly completed. Whereas if the provisional restoration has not been made, the temptation is to hurry this stage often to the detriment of the clinical outcome.

Matrices

Single Units
Wax matrix
This is perhaps one of the simplest and most cost-effective ways of producing a matrix. The method uses softened pink wax moulded around the tooth and allowed to cool and harden. The main advantage of using wax is that alterations to the shape of the crown can be easily achieved (Fig 6-4).

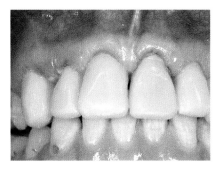

Fig 6-3 There remains a role for long-term, provisional acrylic crowns. Where custom-made they resist stains better than chair-side resin provisional crowns.

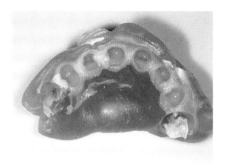

Fig 6-4 Wax matrix, together with the provisional crown.

Silicone matrix
A stiff putty is used to obtain an impression of the tooth (Fig 6-5a,b). Once the preparation is completed the matrix is filled with the provisional material and re-inserted into the mouth. After setting, excess material is removed and the fit of the provisional crown is checked and adjusted accordingly. One major problem with this technique is that changes to the dimensions of the provisional crown are difficult. Rather than attempting to change the silicone impression, it is easier to add composite, without bonding, to the tooth before forming the silicone matrix. The main advantage of using a silicone matrix is that it is dimensionally stable and can be stored between appointments.

Alginate matrix
An alginate matrix requires the use of an impression tray. The difficulty is that changes to the impression are difficult, as the material is friable. In addition, alginate is not dimensionally stable. Despite these inadequacies this technique is commonly used in clinical practice.

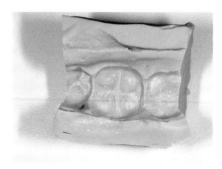 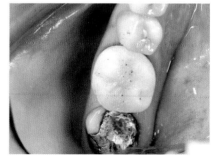

Fig 6-5a A silicone matrix used to make a single provisional crown.

Fig 6-5b The provisional crown formed using the silicone matrix.

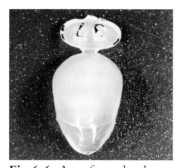

Fig 6-6 A preformed polycarbonate crown.

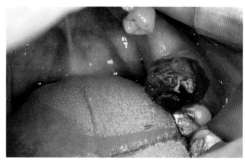

Fig 6-7 Ribbon wax is formed around a prepared tooth from which a temporary crown has been lost.

Preformed crowns

Before the introduction of resin materials, the use of polycarbonate preformed crowns was common (Fig 6-6). They now have limited use and are expensive. The difficulty lies in the inadequacy of the fit of these crowns around the preparation and the need for extensive adjustment, including the need to modify the internal surface with acrylic to adapt them to the preparation. The occlusion is more difficult to adjust.

Other techniques

Occasionally, provisional crowns are lost and there is no matrix. In these circumstances ribbon wax can be adapted to the tooth and an impression taken using either silicone or modellers' wax (Fig 6-7). After adjustments the provisional crown can be formed and fitted. Another way to make a provisional crown is to reline a crown being replaced with cold cure acrylic (Trim, Bosworth) (Fig 6-8).

Multiple Units

In cases in which the shape and size of teeth are to be changed it is important to use a diagnostic wax-up. This gives the patient some understanding of the intended restorations and simplifies the construction of the provisional restorations. The provisional restorations allow the patient to adapt to the shape of the restorations. A diagnostic wax-up (Fig 6-9) can be made from tooth-coloured wax or different coloured waxes. The advantage of using tooth-coloured wax is that it is more realistic for the patient. If the case is especially demanding, alternative mock-ups should be prepared for the patient. This is important when the shape of teeth is being substantially altered to improve appearance. The patient can then select the most pleas-

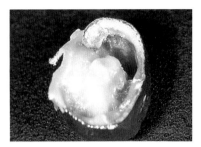

Fig 6-8 An existing crown is used to make a provisional crown. Cold cure acrylic is added to the fit surface of the crown to improve the fit.

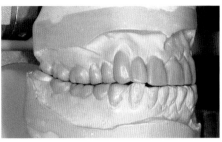

Fig 6-9 Diagnostic wax-up made in tooth-coloured wax provides the patient with an opportunity to better understand and comment on the proposed restorations.

ing tooth form. Additionally, the provisional restorations can be adjusted to refine the final appearance.

Once the diagnostic wax-up has been agreed with the patient, a matrix can be made either in silicone putty or by making a vacuum-formed splint (Fig 6-10 and Fig 6-11) on a replica cast. A silicone impression of the diagnostic wax-up is a simpler, more effective means of producing a matrix.

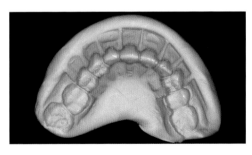

Fig 6-10 A silicone impression taken of the diagnostic wax-up is used to make chair-side provisional crowns.

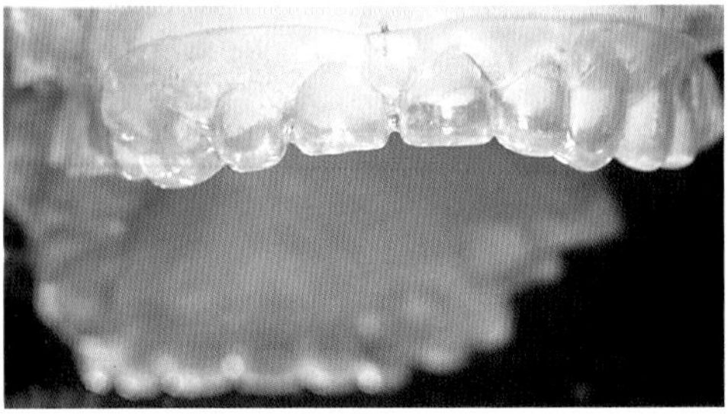

Fig 6-11 Instead of a silicone matrix, the diagnostic cast is replicated and a vacuum-formed matrix is obtained. This matrix is loaded with composite provisional crown material (bis-acryl resin) to obtain good quality, aesthetically pleasing provisional crowns.

Cementing of the Provisional Restorations

The ideal provisional crown cement needs to be a hard cement capable of clinical service over several months, yet simple to remove. For this reason adhesive cements should not be used. Eugenol containing products have the advantage of being adherent without being difficult to remove. A theoretical disadvantage is that the eugenol may subsequently react with a composite luting cement, but this has not been found to be clinically important, provided the cement is completely removed and the preparation thoroughly cleaned and washed. The occlusion should be carefully checked before the provisional crown is cemented. Small deficiencies in the provisional crown can be made good with either more temporary crown and bridge material or a light cured composite.

Tissue Control

For supragingival preparations there is no need for gingival retraction. Provided adequate moisture control can be obtained the need for retraction cord is reduced. Tissues adjacent to subgingival preparations can be managed with ExpaSyl (Kerr UK, Fig 6-12a,b). This material contains aluminium chloride and kaolin. It is gently applied along the gingival margin with an applicator. This material controls bleeding and retracts the tissues. The material is applied at an angle of 45° into the gingival crevice, left in place for about two minutes and then removed by washing. After drying the impression is recorded. The advantage of this product is that it controls bleeding and pro-

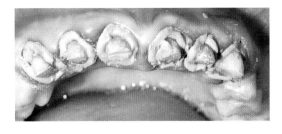

Fig 6-12a ExpaSyl and impression. ExpaSyl causes gingival retraction and prevents bleeding.

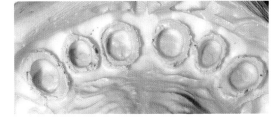

Fig 6-12b Impression of prepared teeth. The margins of the preparations have been recorded. The impression is clinically acceptable.

vides gingival retraction. Another recent innovation is "Magic Foam Cord" (Coltène Whaledent Ltd). This silicone material is syringed around the margins of a preparation in much the same way as ExpaSyl (Fig 6-13a). It is left in place for five minutes, supported by a specially designed compricap (Fig 6-13b). Bubbles are produced as the material sets and expands resulting in retraction of the gingival tissues. Once removed an impression of the preparation can be taken in the normal way.

Subgingival Preparations

The more conventional method to take an impression of a subgingival margin is to displace the adjacent gingival tissues with retraction cord. There are a number of retraction cord systems on the market with a range of diameters available to suit clinical need (Ultradent, West Yorks, England) these cords work by displacing the gingival tissues away from the tooth opening up the gingival sulcus for the impression material. There are a number of ways of recording the impression. The cord can be left in place, and the impression taken. In this technique, it is important to ensure that the cord is not visible around the margin, otherwise the impression will not record

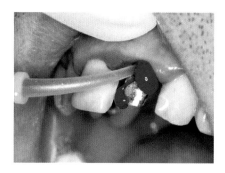

Fig 6-13a Magic foam is used in a similar way to ExpaSyl. This material is syringed around the preparation.

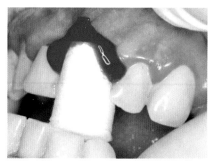

Fig 6-13b A compricap placed over the preparation supports the foam whilst it sets. During the setting reaction the material displaces the gingival tissues exposing the margins of the preparation.

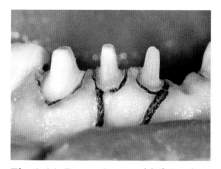

Fig 6-14 Retraction cord left in place and the impression taken over it.

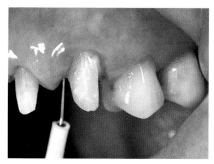

Fig 6-15 Electrosurgery can be used to correct limited gingival overgrowth.

the tooth margin but the cord (Fig 6-14). Another method involves placing one or two cords and then removing one or both of the two strands prior to recording the impression. The disadvantage of these techniques is that removal of the cord may start gingival bleeding which will compromise the impression. This occurs because blood clots form in and around the cord, and are disturbed when the cord is removed. Wetting the cord before removal can reduce, but not completely eliminate this risk. Some manufacturers produce astringent fluids applied before placement of the cord to stop bleeding. Although these can be helpful, they do not control a persistent bleed, which may only be managed by allowing the tissues to heal. This is usually best achieved by placing a good fitting provisional restoration, re-enforcing oral hygiene and having the patient return several days later to record the impression.

Alternatively, bleeding can be reduced by infiltrating a local anaesthetic containing adrenaline into the traumatised area. This causes blanching of the tissues and the vasoconstrictor reduces blood flow temporarily.

Electrosurgery removes localised overgrowth of gingival tissue and controls bleeding (Fig 6-15). Careful and judicious use of electrosurgery can help stem bleeding, but great care is needed to prevent damage to the surrounding vital tissues. The electrosurgery probe should be kept away from the tooth and, in particular, from metal surfaces including posts. Ideally, plastic non-conductive instruments should be used rather than metal instruments. Brief applications to the overgrown tissues avoids overheating and limits iatrogenic damage. For more extensive tissue reduction crown lengthening is indicated.

Impressions

A successful crown is dependant upon a high quality impression of the preparation. The choice of material and tray design may have an impact on accuracy of the impression.

Impression Materials

Probably the most commonly used crown and bridge impression materials are silicones. These can be divided into condensation and addition cured silicones. Condensation cured silicones tend not to be as accurate as addition silicones. This is because alcohol is released as a by-product of the setting reaction of condensation silicones which leads to some shrinkage of the material. Addition cured materials vary in delivery, setting time and viscosity. Some manufacturers have recently claimed that their newer silicone impression materials are hydrophilic, but contamination with blood and saliva remains difficult to overcome. Polyethers remain a popular alternative, and have a proven record, but they suffer some disadvantages relative to addition silicones.

Whichever material is chosen, preparations need to be dry and clear of blood and saliva, with gingival retraction, as appropriate before the impression is recorded. It is worth spending some time drying the teeth to obtain the best impression but excessive drying is to be avoided. Even though silicones and polyether materials claim to be hydrophilic they perform best when the surface is dry. The low viscosity impression materials or single phase materials should be applied to the preparation using a syringe (Fig 6-16). Curved narrow tips allow the material to be syringed into the gingival sulcus. Some operators carefully air blow the impression to distribute the material evenly over the preparation. Care should be taken not to blow too vigorously as this can create air bubbles or displace the material away from the preparation. Whilst this is being done, the impression tray

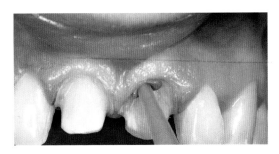

Fig 6-16 The preparation is thoroughly dried and the impression material carefully syringed around the margin.

should be loaded with the corresponding heavy body or putty (if using a silicone) or the same material (if using a monophase material such as a polyether). If moisture control cannot be controlled, an accurate impression is unlikely. In such situations a good, well-fitting provisional restoration, detailed oral hygiene and another appointment is required (Fig 6-17a,b).

The impression is allowed to fully set and then carefully removed by gently breaking the seal with the soft tissue. The impression should be carefully inspected under good lighting to examine for airblows or drags in important areas (Fig 6-18). If a dual phase material is used, it is important to ensure that the low viscosity material is dispensed not only over the preparation but also over the other teeth to ensure an accurate recording of the occlusion. If the low viscosity material starts to set before the putty is seated, the impression should be repeated. The impression is then decontaminated following normal cross infection procedures and dried. All the materials are dimensionally stable in a dry environment. Elastomeric impressions should not be kept in a moist environment.

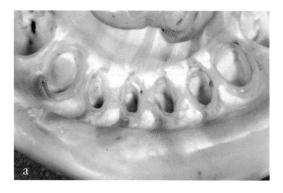

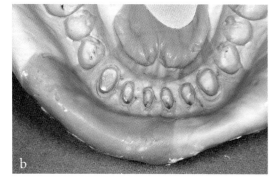

Fig 6-17 (a,b) Impression of the preparation seen in Fig 6-12 (a). The gingival tissues were too inflamed for a successful impression. A week later, during which there was improved oral hygiene, an acceptable impression was obtained.

95

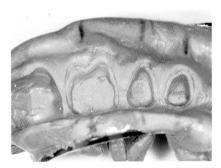

Fig 6-18 The impression is checked for faults. Tears, blow holes and creases indicate an inadequate impression.

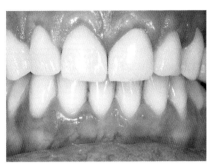

Fig 6-19 The crown is tried in. If acceptable the crown can be cemented.

Choice of Tray

The design and construction, where necessary, of the tray is not particularly important provided it is rigid. There is little advantage in using metal trays over rigid plastic or polycarbonate trays. Some metal trays have so many perforations that a tray adhesive is unnecessary. In most situations, the adhesive is important to ensure that the impression sticks to the tray and does not peel away. This is most likely to occur on withdrawal of the impression from the mouth, in particular, if the impression is overextended into undercut areas.

Bonnets

It is difficult to achieve a satisfactory impression of multiple preparations. In these situations "bonnets" made of Duralay (Reliance Dental) can help to achieve an accurate impression. Individual bonnets or copings are made on stone dies cast from accurate impressions. With the bonnets in place, a working impression is obtained to record the interrelationship of the preparations. This is sometimes referred to as a "pick-up" impression.

Interocclusal Records

In most cases, provided there is an obvious intercuspal position (ICP) and this can be readily located on the working casts, an interocclusal record is unnecessary. An interocclusal record is, however, important when the ICP cannot be easily located, and where there is a planned increase in the vertical dimension, or when multiple restorations are constructed. There are a number of materials available. Whichever material is chosen, it is important that the casts can be accurately relocated. Some manufacturers have produced silicone occlusal registration materials which are hard and quick setting. These materials can be carved with a sharp knife or scalpel to remove any excess. Other materials include wax rims refined with zinc oxide eugenol impression material. It is important before articulating the casts that any artefacts, such as airblows, are removed as these cause interferences (see Chapter 9).

Fitting Crowns

The first stage is to check if the restoration fits the laboratory working cast. If not minor adjustments can be made. If the crown does not fit the model, the crown should be rejected and a new impression taken. Common problems (Fig 6-19) with the fit of restorations on working dies include:

- over-trimming of the margin resulting in a negative fit
- tight contacts between the teeth, which should be adjusted in the mouth
- incomplete contact areas, which normally indicate starting again with a new impression
- blemishes on the fit surface of the crown, which should be removed as they interfere with seating.

When satisfied with the fit of the restoration on the die, the restoration should be tried-in in the mouth, subsequent to removal of the provisional restoration and careful cleaning of the preparation. Particular attention is required to ensure that no temporary cement remains, as this may prevent the restoration fully seating when tried-in. Other common reasons for a restoration not fully seating at try-in include:
- tight proximal contacts
- soft tissue getting caught between the restoration and the preparation
- blemishes on the fitting surface of the restoration.

The procedure for checking the occlusion is discussed in Chapter 9. Chairside adjustments to the occlusion of crowns are normally guided by articulating paper (Fig 6-20). Finally, all the adjusted surfaces should be polished.

Polishing the Crown

After the final adjustments, the occlusal surface may be rough and should be polished prior to cementation. There is an advantage in requesting sandblasted metal occlusal surfaces for metal-based crowns. This process has the advantage that polishing is made simpler but also facilitates seeing occlusal contacts highlighted by articulating paper. In the mandible most patients prefer a ceramic surface. Whichever surface is chosen, polishing is impor-

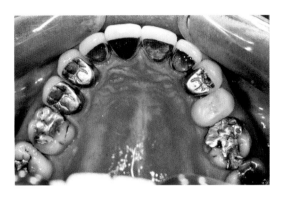

Fig 6-20 The articulating paper marks indicating even occlusal contact on the crowns and adjacent teeth.

tant to limit wear to the opposing tooth or crown. Polishing metals is straightforward, and can be done at the chair-side. Porcelain can also be polished at the chair-side rather than re-glazed. The surface finish produced by diamond impregnated polishing wheels can be as smooth as a reglaze. The disadvantage of reglazing is that the surface of the porcelain may slump during glazing and more occlusal adjustment may be needed. Wherever possible, polishing should be undertaken on the working model rather than with the restoration handheld.

Final Cementation

After adjustments and polishing, but before cementation, it is important to have the patient approve the restoration and agree to it being cemented. Do not be tempted to rush this stage as the patient needs to feel ownership of the restoration. Crowns can be cemented with provisional cements to confirm patient acceptance and intended function. In such situations it is important to use a weak or weakened mix of a provisional cement.

The choice of luting cement is personal, as there is little scientific evidence to suggest that any one material is more effective than another for conventional preparations. For teeth with short clinical crowns the use of a composite resin luting cement with a dentine bonding agent is recommended together with modification to the fitting surface of the restoration to encourage micromechanical interlock, if not bonding. Although glass-ionomer cements bond to teeth, they are weaker than composites. After fitting the crown, great care has to be taken to ensure that all excess luting cement has been removed. Finally, instruct the patient on oral hygiene and make a review appointment.

Most resin-based cements include a dentine bonding agent to improve the bond strength to dentine. This is particularly important with crowns as most of the tissue exposed during preparation is dentine. In most conventional situations, key issues are a careful clinical technique and the use of the material according to the manufacturer's instructions. The advantage of capsulated cements is that a consistent mix is assured each time. Many glass-ionomer cements are packaged this way. Zinc phosphate remains a useful and reliable cement, provided it is mixed appropriately and carefully handled.

Whatever cement is chosen it is important to follow the manufacturer's directions to ensure an optimum outcome. Once the cement is set, carefully remove excess with a probe, working in an apical direction rather than coronally, which might lead to unseating the restoration. Clear the contact points with dental floss and then finally check the occlusion before dismissing the patient. If photographs are required, it is better to take these at a review appointment or prior to cementation. This is because some degree of gingival bleeding always occurs during cementation and it is difficult to remove all cement debris from the field of view.

Choice of Cement

Types of Luting Cement
There are a number of luting cements, each with advantages and disadvantages. Commonly used types of luting cement include:
• zinc oxide and eugenol
• zinc phosphate
• zinc polycarboxylate
• glass-ionomer
• resin-modified glass-ionomer
• resin-based luting cements.

Zinc Oxide and Eugenol
Zinc oxide and eugenol luting cement should be used as a temporary cement. Its compressive strength and solubility makes it unsuitable as a permanent cement. Its main advantage is its obtundant effect on the pulp dentine complex. If used with a restoration which will eventually be resin-bonded, care is required to completely remove the zinc oxide and eugenol cement and to clean the surfaces to be bonded to preclude the resin lute being compromised by eugenol – an essential oil.

Zinc Phosphate

Zinc phosphate luting cements have a long and tried history and are still commonly used due to their ease of use, reliablility and low cost. The cement is presented as a zinc oxide powder with an aqueous solution of phosphoric acid. Final properties of the cement depend upon the ratio in which the components are mixed. For example, compressive strength and resistance to dissolution increases with the proportion of powder. These properties are not, however, acquired for up to 24 hours. Care should be taken by the patient to protect the setting cement during this period by avoiding excessive loading. Although an increase in the powder to liquid ratio improves the physical properties, it also produces a more viscous mix.

The working and setting time of zinc phosphate can be quick. Various techniques can be used to delay the setting time, including:
- slowly adding small amounts of powder to the liquid (slaking)
- the working time can be extended by mixing the cement over a large surface area using a cooled glass slab.

The main disadvantage of zinc phosphate cement is the early acidity of the freshly mixed cement which can cause sensitivity. This sensitivity is transient, lasting only a few hours. Sensitivity is likely to be worse in extensively prepared teeth – particularly if a thin mix of the cement has been used as the pH tends to remain lower for longer. In certain cases, it may be necessary to anaesthetise the tooth to cement a crown with zinc phosphate. Zinc phosphate cement remains a cost-effective, useful luting cement for conventional indirect restorations, placed on both vital and non-vital teeth.

Zinc Polycarboxylate

Most zinc polycarboxylate luting cements are presented as a powder and liquid. The powder consists of zinc oxide with a small proportion of magnesium oxide and the liquid is polyacrylic acid. Some manufacturers freeze dry the acid and add it to the powder, in which case the powder is mixed with sterile water. When initially mixed to the manufacturer's recommended powder to liquid ratio, the cement appears thick; however, because of its thixotropic/pseudoplastic nature, it flows when under pressure. The temptation to make a thinner mix should therefore be avoided.

Like zinc phosphate cement polycarboxylate cements are acidic when mixed, however, the pH rises rapidly as the material sets and the potential for sensitivity is reduced. Care should be taken when using zinc polycarboxylate cements as they have a relatively fast setting reaction, leading to increasing viscosity and the potential to prevent the restoration fully seating.

It is suggested that the difficulties with the handling of zinc polycarboxylate cements outweigh its advantages and it should be reserved for the cementation of metal based restorations and avoided in preparations in close proximity to the pulp.

Glass-ionomers

Glass–ionomer cements are popular luting cements. They are mixed as a powder and liquid. The powder is an aluminium fluorosilicate glass and the liquid, a relatively weak polyalkenoic acid. Like zinc polycarboxylate cements the acid is sometimes freeze–dried and incorporated into the powder. It is reconstituted by mixing with water. The powder to liquid ratio is critical. Alterations to the ratio affects working time and viscosity and, in general results in an inferior mix. To ensure consistent and optimum properties, some manufacturers produce encapsulated materials.

Once mixed, the material remains at a constant viscosity for sufficient time to allow accurate seating. The initial low pH might cause sensitivity, but it is usually mild and transient. Once set, the material achieves higher compressive strength than zinc phosphate and zinc polycarboxylate cements; however, it is more likely to deform in high stress regions due to a lower modulus of elasticity.

The main benefits of this material are adhesion to tooth tissue and the gradual leaching of fluoride ions. Numerous claims have been made about the fluoride leaching and the potential for reducing secondary caries. The amount of fluoride released is unlikely to have an effect on secondary caries. All glass-ionomer luting cements are susceptible to dehydration and dissolution. To prevent such adverse effects light cured bonding resin may be applied over the restoration margins. Nevertheless, this resin will be lost within a day or two of placement.

In general, glass-ionomer luting cements perform well in the luting of well-fitting metal and metal–ceramic crowns.

Resin-modified Glass-ionomer

Unlike restorative resin-modified glass-ionomers which can be light-cured, luting versions of these cements are chemically or dual cured. The cement sets conventionally by an acid base reaction, and by polymerisation of the methacrylate side groups. The resin component allows the luting cement to bond to both tooth tissues and composite. Compared with conventional glass–ionomer luting cements, resin modified glass–ionomer cements have a reduced solubility and increased compressive and tensile strengths. These qualities make resin-modified glass-ionomer luting systems ideal for cementing metal-based, indirect restorations. These cements should not, however, be used for ceramic restorations as they undergo hygroscopic expansion. This can potentially lead to fracture of all-ceramic crowns, in particular, when a resin-modified glass-ionomer core has been placed.

Resin-based Luting Cements
Resin–based luting cements are either dual or light cured. These cements tend to have a much lower filler content than resin–based restorative materials. This results in a lower viscosity allowing complete seating of the restoration with a thin lute thickness. The light cured cements can only be used in conjunction with veneer restorations. Inlays, onlays and crowns need to be bonded using a dual-cured cement.

When cementing all–ceramic crowns, the preparation and core should be etched and the appropriate dentine bonding agent applied to the tooth. Resins will not bond to the fit surface of ceramic restorations without surface roughening. Sandblasting the fit surface with 50μm alumina will roughen the surface, however greater roughness is achieved by etching with hydrofluoric acid. Hydrofluoric acid is extremely corrosive and must be handled with extreme care.

Because composite resins do not bond directly to ceramics a silane coupling agent is needed to achieve the bond. This bipolar molecule bonds to the ceramic surface and the methacrylate end of the resin cement. A number of chemically adhesive resin luting cements have been developed in which the resin is modified with a phosphate monomer (Panavia 21, Kuraray Co) or 4-META (4-methacryloxyethyl trimellitate anhydride) (C&B Superbond, Sun Medical Co) to enable it to bond to sandblasted metal.

Summary

Stages in Crown Preparations

Single Restorations Without the Need for a Diagnostic Wax-up

The stages following preoperative assessment, including radiographic and vitality tests for single units, are as follows:

- Take shade of tooth
- Administer local anaesthesia
- Obtain matrix of the tooth whilst anaesthesia is taking effect
- Prepare tooth for crown
- Soft tissue management
- Make provisional restoration
- Take impression
- Fit provisional restoration.

Multiple Restorations with Diagnostic Wax-ups

In contrast, the stages for multiple restorations following preoperative assessment, including radiographic, vitality tests and study casts, are as follows:

- Make diagnostic wax-up on articulated study casts
- Patient acceptance of the proposed shape and shade of teeth
- Administer local anaesthesia
- Obtain matrix from the diagnostic wax-up
- Prepare the teeth
- Soft tissue management
- Make provisional restorations
- Take impression
- Record intra-occlusal record
- Facebow recording
- Fit provisional restorations.

Cementation of Definitive Crowns

- Remove provisional restorations
- Remove remaining cement from preparations
- Try-in crowns
- Adjust crown as necessary
- Clean and isolate the prepared teeth
- Clean and, where necessary, modify or prime the fitting surface of the restoration
- Dispense, mix and apply the selected luting cement in strict accordance with manufacturer's directions
- Wait for cement to set and remove excess

- Give the patient oral hygiene and other instructions as may be necessary
- Review crown within 1–2 weeks to check for patient satisfaction.

Above all else, it is to be remembered that no cement system can compensate for inadequate, poorly planned preparations and ill-fitting restorations. Most cement failures are a consequence of either poor technique or too much being expected of the cement.

Chapter 7
Managing the Occlusion

Aim

The aim of this chapter is to review those aspects of occlusion of relevance to provision of crowns.

Objective

After this chapter the reader will understand the importance of occlusion in making crowns.

Introduction

The term occlusion conjures up an image of a static relationship with the upper and lower teeth in contact. Whilst this relationship is important, the way in which the teeth move over one another in excursive movements is equally important. The occlusion and articulation of the teeth should be in harmony with the temporomandibular joints and muscles of mastication. This does not mean that dentitions should be restored to a stylised version of a balanced occlusion. By virtue of periodontal mechanoreceptors and proprioceptors patients adapt to considerable variations in the "ideal" occlusion. Patients also adapt to changes made to their occlusion. However, this adaptive capacity cannot be quantified or predicted. If changes are made to the occlusion, these should be in a planned and well controlled way.

Most indirect restorations should be made to conform to the existing occlusion in such a way that they are functional and do not introduce occlusal interferences – the so-called "conformative approach" to restorative dentistry. When more advanced restorative work is undertaken and the occlusal relationship is altered; this is called a "reorganised approach".

Intercuspal Position (ICP)

When a patient is asked to close, the teeth will normally be brought into intercuspal position (ICP). This occurs as a result of a learnt pattern of closure, influenced by afferent feedback from periodontal mechanoreceptors. The ICP is the jaw relationship when the upper and lower teeth are in maximum intercuspation (Fig 7-1). When the jaw is in this position, it is important to evaluate the occlusal vertical dimension and whether the occlusion is stable.

Occlusal Vertical Dimension

The occlusal vertical dimension is a measure of the height of the occlusion when the teeth are in the ICP. The occlusal vertical dimension is of particular importance in patients with extensive tooth wear who are being considered for operative intervention. It might be anticipated that extensive tooth wear would be accompanied by a reduction in occlusal vertical dimension. This is not usually the case if the tooth wear has been gradual, because dentoalveolar compensation maintains the occlusal vertical dimension. Frequently, tooth wear is localised to the palatal surfaces of the upper anterior teeth. The resulting dentoalveolar compensation leads to overeruption of the lower incisors to maintain tooth contact (Fig 7-2). In these situations the result is upper anterior teeth with shortened clinical crowns which, if reduced further for conventional full coverage crowns, can lead to nonretentive preparations. The management of the occlusion in such situations is described later in this book.

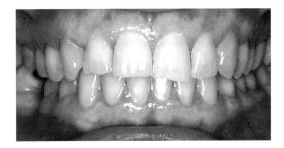

Fig 7-1 Patient closed in the intercuspal position (ICP).

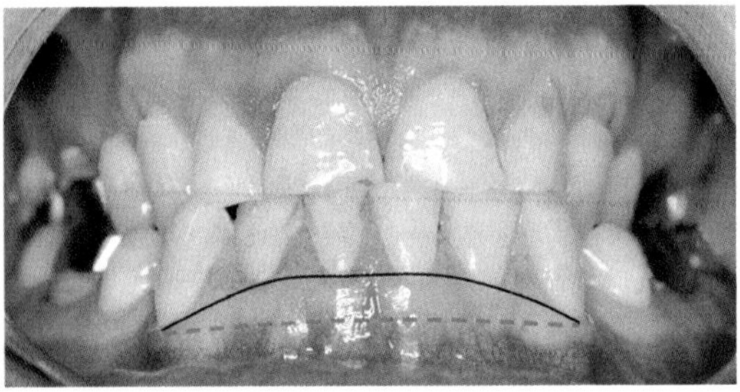

Fig 7-2 Localised tooth wear has caused dentoalveolar compensation with maintained tooth contact as the teeth became shortened. The gingival level in the lower anterior region has risen and become bowed with the compensation.

(The blue dotted line at the bottom is the original gingival level and the top purple line is the gingival level following tooth wear and dentoalveolar compensation)

Stable Occlusion

A stable occlusion is one in which there is no potential for overeruption, drifting or tilting of the teeth. In the patient in Fig 7–3a–g, early loss of the lower first permanent molar led to mesial tilting of the lower second molar and overeruption of the upper first molar as this tooth was unopposed. This led to an occlusal interference. Therefore, if teeth are extracted, it is important to remember to assess whether the occlusion is unstable and, if so, to consider early replacement of the lost teeth with a fixed or removable prosthesis. If a decision is made not to replace teeth, then monitoring of tooth movement can be carried out with the aid of dated study casts. This allows planned management of the occlusion (Fig 7–3b–g).

Terminal Hinge Axis and Retruded Contact Position (RCP)

The terminal hinge axis position is where the condyles of the mandible are in their most superior and posterior position in the glenoid fossa. If an imaginary axis is drawn through the centre of each condyle (Fig 7–4a–c), pure rotation of the mandible occurs for the first 20 mm on opening (Fig 7–4b). The first tooth contact, when the mandible is in the terminal hinge axis position, is called the retruded contact position (RCP) or centric relation. In over 90% of dentate patients RCP and ICP (centric occlusion) do not coincide. There is usually an anterior and superior slide of approximately 2 mm between the two positions (Fig 7–4b and Fig 7–5a–c). When adopting a conformative approach, it is important that restorations do not interfere with this slide.

The relevance of these positions becomes apparent when adopting a reorganised approach to the occlusion. Examples include: increasing the occlusal vertical dimension, restoring the occlusal surface of a tooth with a RCP contact, and when creating space for full coverage restorations on short clinical crowns in the upper anterior region.

Lateral Excursions

In lateral excursions, the side to which the mandible moves is called the working side and the contralateral side is the non-working side.

Working Side
The guidance on the working side dictates the downward movement of the mandible in lateral excursion. Guidance on the working side is typically, either canine guided or group function.

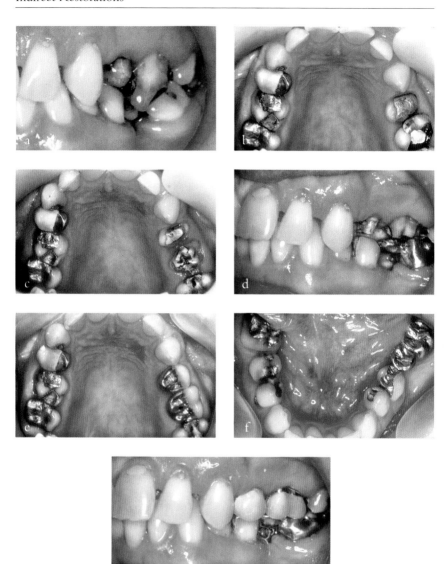

Fig 7-3 (a–g) Early loss of the lower molar tooth has led to an unstable occlusion, with tilting, drifting and overeruption of teeth into the space (a). To eliminate the resultant occlusal interference and create an acceptable occlusion, the upper first permanent molar was elective root treated as extensive occlusal reduction was required (b). This allowed preparation of the teeth for metal–ceramic crowns (c and d) and placement of a fixed movable bridge in the lower arch (e and f) and the completed restoration (g).

Fig 7-4 (a-c) An axis drawn through the head of each condyle is shown in Fig 7-4a. When the condyles are in the most posterior and superior position in the glenoid fossa, the mandible is said to be in the terminal hinge axis position (THA). If an imaginary stylus is placed between the lower central incisor teeth and viewed laterally (Fig 7-4b) the first 20 mm or so of opening involves rotation of the mandible or hinge opening (HO) around the THA.

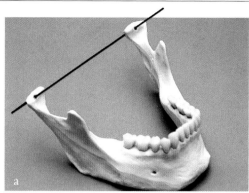

On further opening, the condyles slide downwards and forwards onto the articular eminence until maximum opening (MO) is reached. The first tooth contact when the mandible is in the THA position is called the retruded contact position (RCP). In most dentate patients (>90%) there is an anterior and upward slide into intercuspal position (ICP). On protrusion the anterior teeth guide the mandibular movement - so called anterior guidance (A).

The degree of guidance will depend on the incisal relationship (Fig 7-4c). The teeth remain in contact in maximum protrusion (P). The movement of the mandible dictated by the teeth (RCP-ICP-A-P) and the musculature, ligaments and skeleton (RCP-HO-MO-P) traced in the sagittal plane (Fig 7-4b) is called Posselt's envelope of movement.

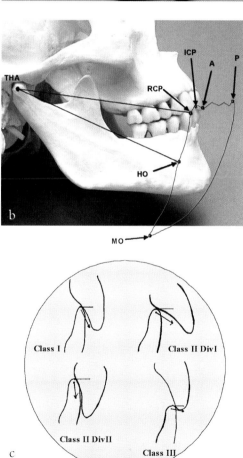

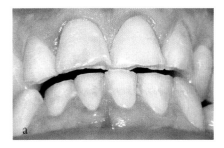
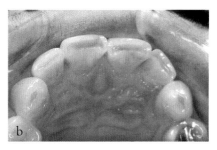

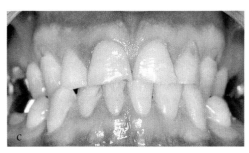

Fig 7-5 (a–c) This figure shows the same patient seen in Fig 7-2. When the mandible is in the terminal hinge axis position, horizontal space is created between the upper and lower incisor teeth (a). The occlusal view (b) shows obvious wear facets indicating the ICP slide position when the teeth are in edge-to-edge contact (c).

Non-working Side

The non-working side is frequently overlooked when placing indirect restorations. It has been suggested by some clinicians that non-working contacts should be avoided as they are associated with temporomandibular joint disorders. This claim must be treated with caution as many patients have asymptomatic non-working side contacts. When placing restorations, it is prudent not to introduce new non-working contacts.

As the mandible moves to the right, for example, the non-working left condyle moves forwards, downwards and inwards in an arch pivoted around the working condyle (Fig 7-6). On the non-working side, the condylar inclination dictates the degree of downward movement. In patients with a shallow condylar inclination, the downward movement of the mandible on the non-working side is small and the potential for introducing non-working side contacts is high. To avoid this, it is important not to provide restorations with prominent cusps with steep inclines.

Canine Guidance

When the opposing surfaces of the upper and lower canine teeth guide the mandible to the working side in lateral excursions, it is termed canine

Fig 7-6 (a,b) In protrusion the condyles move downwards and forwards from the glenoid fossa onto the articular eminence. The angle this makes with the horizontal when the patient is sitting upright is called the condylar inclination (a). In lateral excursion, the non-working condyle not only moves down onto the articular eminence, it also moves medially. As viewed from above, the angle this makes with the sagittal plane is called the Bennett angle (b). Also in lateral excursion there is a bodily sideways movement of the mandible, which can be measured on the working side condyle and this is termed Bennett movement (b).

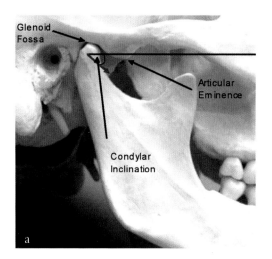

As seen in Fig 7-4, if the tracings of an imaginary stylus between the lower incisors are viewed in the horizontal plane (outlined in red in Fig 7-4b), when the mandible moves into lateral excursion there is a rotation around the working condyle. The red outline in Fig 7-4b is sometimes referred to as a Gothic Arch tracing, linking the points of maximum left and right lateral excursion with maximum protrusion.

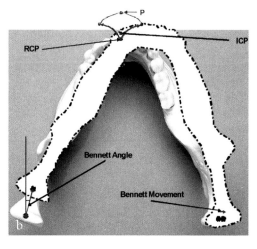

guidance (Fig 7-7). Prominent canine guidance will cause the occlusal surfaces of mandibular teeth to disclude, reducing the likelihood of non-working side contacts developing.

Restoring the Canine

If a canine tooth is restored, a decision needs to be taken whether to reproduce the canine guidance. In general, restorations should restore the guidance, unless the canine is root filled and has a post retained core with a guarded prognosis.

111

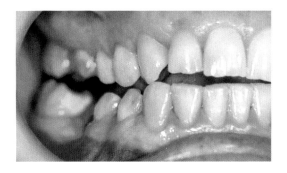

Fig 7-7 In right lateral excursion this patient has canine guidance.

Restoring Posterior Teeth

Restoring posterior teeth in patients with canine guidance is relatively simple. In lateral excursions, the canines guide the mandible towards the working side, separating the posterior teeth. In these situations, the ICP contacts in new restorations are critical (Fig 7-8a-c). For single posterior crowns in patients with an easily reproducible ICP, only handheld articulation is necessary. When the occlusal surfaces of multiple posterior teeth are to be restored, and in cases in which it will be difficult for the technician to keep

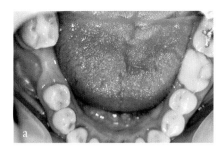

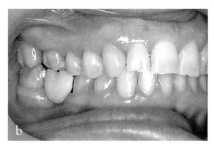

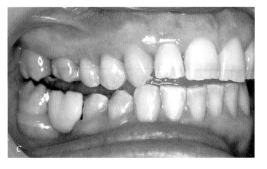

Fig 7-8 (a-c) Patient seen in Fig 7-1 requires a minimal preparation prepared bridge incorporating the mesioocclusal cavity in the second molar tooth (a). There is a large occlusal area to check and potentially adjust in ICP (b), but in lateral excursion posterior disclusion means no further adjustment will be necessary (c).

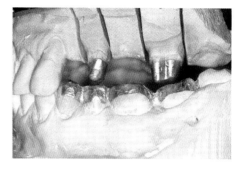

Fig 7-9 This patient had a four unit bridge in the upper left quadrant which needed replacement. The patient had canine guidance and the models were articulated on a simple hinge articulator to stabilise them. ICP contacts were carefully checked, but little if no occlusal adjustment was needed as the posterior teeth discluded in lateral excursion.

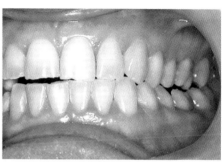

Fig 7-10 This patient (seen in Fig 7-1) had group function in left lateral excursion and required a core and crown placement on the lower left first permanent molar. This is potentially more difficult than placement of the bridge in the lower right quadrant as ICP contacts and contacts in lateral excursion have to be checked and carefully adjusted.

the casts stable (Fig 7-9), articulation on a simple hinge articulator or semi-adjustable articulator is recommended. When multiple teeth are involved, a semiadjustable articulator is essential.

Group Function

The term group function is used when two or more pairs of teeth guide the mandible in lateral excursions (Fig 7-10). In this situation there may be simultaneous contact between anterior and posterior teeth.

Difficulties
Restoring the occlusal surfaces of posterior teeth is more difficult in patients with group function than canine guidance. In addition to ICP contacts, the contact between the guiding teeth needs to be maintained during excursive movements. When making more than one crown, semiadjustable articulators help to reproduce the working side contacts and ensure that non-working side contacts are avoided. Patients with extensive tooth wear may have group function as a result of shallow or negligible cuspal inclines. In lateral excursions, there is little downward movement of the mandible and on the

non-working side care has to be taken not to introduce non-working side interferences.

Anterior Guidance
The relationship between opposing incisors will govern the anterior guidance in protrusive and laterotrusive movements (Fig 7-4c). In Class I and Class II division II incisal relationships, anterior guidance causes posterior disclusion, influencing the complexity of restoring anterior and posterior teeth. For example, a Class II division II incisal relationship may cause great technical difficulty when restoring anterior teeth but makes the construction of posterior restorations relatively simple. For patients with Class II division I incisal relationship, the situation is reversed.

Reproducing Anterior and Canine Guidance (Fig 7-11a-g)
Not every canine or anterior tooth requiring an indirect restoration poses technical difficulties. In contrast, restoring anterior teeth with crowns in a patient with a Class II division II incisal relationship includes the challenge that the palatal contour of the upper anterior crown is technically demanding. The increased overbite and reduced overjet means that the palatal surfaces of the retroclined upper incisors are tightly adapted to the incisal edges of the lower incisors. In such situations, it may be helpful to make an incisal guidance table on the articulator, which should be semiadjustable (Fig 7-11). With the casts mounted in the ICP, ensure that the incisal pin on the articulator touches the incisal guidance table. In lateral and protrusive movements the incisal pin rises off the table, guided by the shape of the palatal surfaces of the upper anterior teeth. The movement of the pin can be recorded by placing freshly mixed cold cured acrylic resin on the incisal guidance table and performing lateral and protrusive movements. The incisal pin moulds the setting acrylic into a crescent shaped ramp, forming an incisal guidance

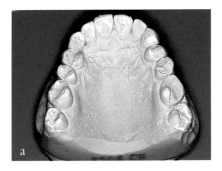

Fig 7-11 (a) *Reproducing anterior guidance* This patient presented with a four unit fixed-bridge replacing the missing upper right canine, with linked retainers on the upper right incisor and a retainer on the upper right first premolar. The bridge had been in place for 22 years, however, the ceramic had fractured distally on the upper right first premolar leading to food packing and caries.

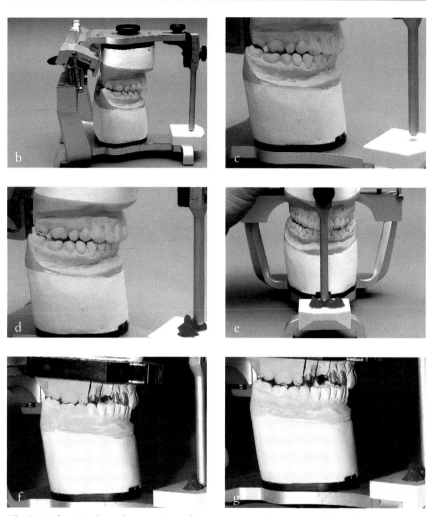

Fig 7-11 (b-g) In lateral excursion, the anterior guidance needed to be reproduced in the replacement bridge. Study casts including the original bridge were articulated on a semiadjustable articulator (b), and lateral excursive movements reproduced, raising the incisal guidance pin off the incisal table of the articulator (c). Cold cure acrylic was placed on the incisal table and the movements repeated whilst the acrylic set (d). All excursive movements, including protrusion (e) were reproduced in the same way creating a so-called *custom-formed incisal guidance table*. At the next appointment the bridge was removed, impressions taken and a working model mounted on the same articulator (f). Excursive movements were guided by the custom-formed incisal guidance table (g), allowing the technician to wax-up the substructure of the bridge to conform to the guidance of the original bridge.

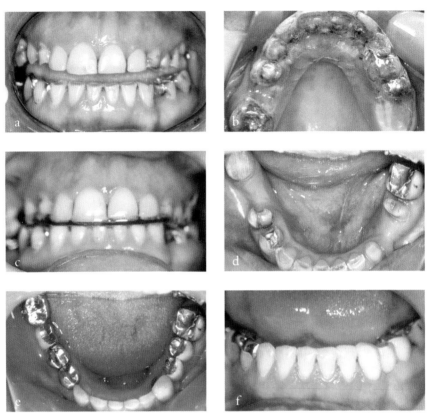

Fig 7-12 (a-f) A reorganised approach to restoring a patient's dentition with tooth wear. This patient presented with an extensively restored dentition, missing posterior teeth, generalised tooth wear and failing restorations, including the ceramic veneers placed on the upper incisor teeth (a). Initially, study casts were articulated and a full diagnostic wax-up made on a semiadjustable articulator using an RCP interocclusal record. The incisal pin on the articulator was raised 3 mm to provide sufficient space to restore the anterior teeth (Fig 7-4b).

The patient's tolerance of this increase in occlusal vertical dimension was assessed using a clear, hard acrylic splint (Michigan splint) (b and c). This also helped to eliminate occlusal interferences and made recording of the terminal hinge axis position easier. The posterior teeth in the lower arch were prepared for crowns and bridge retainers (d) with a minimum of occlusal reduction to preserve crown height and retention. The increased occlusal vertical dimension created was sufficient to place direct composite restorations to the lower anterior teeth (e and f). Placement of the posterior indirect restorations and placement of the composites must be done at the same visit to prevent overeruption of the anterior teeth.

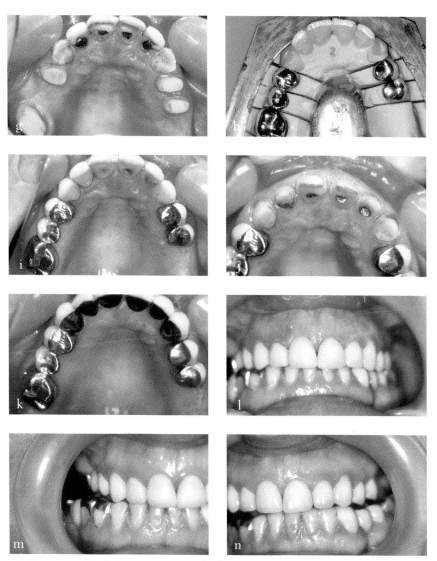

Fig 7-12 (g-n) Similarly in the upper arch, the posterior teeth were prepared for crowns and a bridge (g), and the restorations made on a model together with the waxed up anterior teeth (h), ensuring that anterior guidance could be created in the definitive anterior crowns. The posterior restorations were cemented and composite placed on the palatal surface of the upper anterior teeth to preserve the occlusal clearance created (i). At a later appointment the upper anterior teeth were prepared (j) and the desired anterior guidance, created in the diagnostic wax-up, was reproduced in the crowns (k-n).

117

table. The custom-formed incisal guidance table allows the reproduction of the shape of the palatal surfaces of the upper incisors in the construction of the crowns.

Conformative vs. Reorganised Approach

Individual single cast restorations to be placed in an otherwise sound dental arch are constructed to conform to the existing occlusal scheme. In contrast, when the dentition has suffered wear or substantial damage, a new occlusal scheme is needed. A reorganised occlusion is normally restored to the terminal hinge axis position (Fig 7-12a-n) – the most reproducible jaw relationship.

A Michigan splint can be used to assess the patient's tolerance of an increased occlusal vertical dimension. It also disengages the occlusion, disrupting any conditioned paths of closure, allowing the terminal hinge axis to be recorded (Fig 7-12b,c). In cases in which it is difficult to guide the jaw into the terminal hinge axis position, the splint may need to be adjusted on more than one occasion, allowing the terminal hinge axis position to be readily recorded.

In full arch reconstructions there is some debate as to which teeth should be restored first; the anterior teeth to establish the shape and size of the teeth and the anterior guidance or the posterior teeth to establish the vertical dimension. There is no evidence in the literature to suggest which approach should be adopted. The decision should be based on clinical circumstances. For the patient illustrated in Fig 7-12, the posterior teeth were restored first to establish the vertical dimension and composites used to provide anterior guidance. The posterior restorations were made on a working model using a diagnostic wax-up of the anterior teeth, ensuring the selected anterior guidance. Conversely, restoring the anterior teeth first allows the shape of the teeth in the smile line to be determined first, prior to restoring the posterior teeth. For most people, the appearance of the anterior teeth is critical. Therefore, even when a diagnostic wax-up is used to guide the shape of the anterior teeth, provisional crowns should be used to ensure the patient is satisfied with their shape.

Further Reading

Klineberg I, Jagger R. Occlusion and Clinical Practice: an Evidence-based approach. London: Wright, 2004.

Chapter 8
Short Clinical Crowns

Aim

The aim of this chapter is to review the problems associated with short clinical crowns and learn how to manage them.

Objectives

After reading this chapter the reader will appreciate the difficulties of managing teeth with short clinical crowns and understand how to overcome these difficulties.

Introduction

A difficult clinical treatment planning problem is the restoration of the short clinical crown. The principal problem associated with a short clinical crown is the retention of the restoration within the existing vertical space. Difficulties with short clinical crowns may be limited to single teeth, localised to a few teeth or be part of a more generalised problem. Management depends on the number of teeth involved and the vertical height of the existing teeth. Traditional management of teeth with short clinical crowns involves preparation of near parallel walls with slots or grooves to maximise the retention. In extreme situations, elective root treatment is advocated to gain additional retention from the root canal. Adhesive resins and techniques for the management of dento-alveolar compensation have simplified the treatment of the short clinical crown.

Single Teeth

The common causes of short clinical crowns on single teeth are:
• trauma
• replacement crowns
• loss of crown height and overeruption.

Trauma
Trauma can result in substantial loss of enamel and dentine. Provided sufficient vertical space exists and a provisional restoration is placed to prevent

overeruption of the opposing teeth, the complexity of the restoration depends on the amount of tooth tissue remaining and the status of the pulp. In most cases, the restoration is conventional and the management follows well established restorative techniques. In more extreme cases, the tooth may become non-vital and a root filling with or without a post retained crown is indicated to restore the tooth.

Replacement Crowns

Replacement crowns are common because of marginal caries, changes to the appearance of crowns and adjacent teeth, recession of the gingival tissues and mechanical failure. Situations may arise when a replacement crown becomes difficult once the existing crown is removed and the underlying tooth examined. For example, caries removal might produce subgingival margins or a short preparation requiring a core build-up in direct composite. An alternative is to incorporate the deficiency into the crown preparation (Fig 8-1 and Fig 8-2). The advantage of this technique is that the cement lute links the tooth to the crown directly, rather than being sandwiched between the crown and another restorative material.

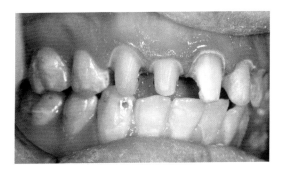

Fig 8-1 This patient with fluorosis needed anterior crowns. Existing restorations were removed from the anterior teeth, but not replaced.

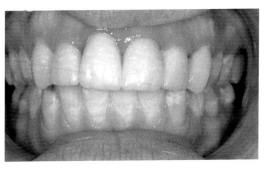

Fig 8-2 The completed crowns.

Loss of Crown and Overeruption of Teeth

A crown lost as a consequence of a cement failure may cause the overeruption of the opposing tooth and closure of the vertical space which accommodated the lost crown. The result is a short clinical crown in functional occlusion with the opposing tooth. This overeruption needs to be managed either orthodontically or by elective crown lengthening surgery. The former does not involve further occlusal reduction and is simpler to undertake. Apical re-positioning of the gingival margin necessitates further occlusal reduction and can lead to pulpal exposure, necessitating elective endodontic treatment.

An alternative option to reverse the loss of space is to place direct composite onto the occlusal surface of the tooth, intentionally making the restoration high. For example, Fig 8-3a, 8-3b and 8-3c show what can happen when a tooth prepared for a conventional metal-ceramic crown lost its provisional crown. The prepared tooth overerupted and made contact with the opposing tooth, producing a short clinical crown. Placing a thin veneer of composite on the occlusal surface, with a thickness to match the amount of vertical space needed, reversed the overeruption within a few weeks and allowed a replacement crown to be made. If the time between crown loss and overeruption is short, then the time taken for the reversal will normally be correspondingly short.

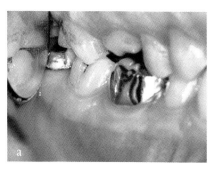

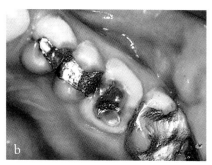

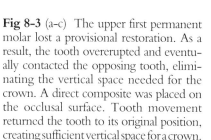

Fig 8-3 (a-c) The upper first permanent molar lost a provisional restoration. As a result, the tooth overerupted and eventually contacted the opposing tooth, eliminating the vertical space needed for the crown. A direct composite was placed on the occlusal surface. Tooth movement returned the tooth to its original position, creating sufficient vertical space for a crown.

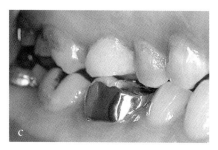

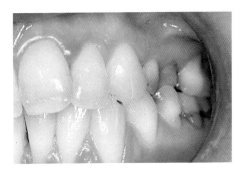

Fig 8-4 Providing a crown on the upper second premolar will involve short preparations and a gingival contour which will not conform to the sagittal plane.

One problem with overerupting teeth is the simultaneous movement of the gingival margin. Reversing overeruption normally results in the movement of the gingival margin back to its original position with a good aesthetic outcome. Crown lengthening apically repositions the gingival margin and may not achieve a satisfactory result. Accepting a short crown often results in an unacceptable gingival contour on anterior teeth (Fig 8-4). This tends to be unacceptable to the patient.

Surgical crown lengthening increases the vertical height of teeth, but is an unpleasant experience for the patient. The surgical repositioning of the gingival margin apically increases the crown length, but further occlusal reduction is necessary to provide space for the crown (Fig 8-5a,b).

When assessing the impact of the surgery it is important to note the radiographic position of the pulp. It may also be prudent to practise the crown preparation on study casts. Trial preparations aid in planning surgery. If the amount of space needed for occlusal reduction results in pulpal exposure, crown lengthening may be inappropriate. Other problems with crown lengthening surgery include dentinal sensitivity and the formation of an uneven gingival contour with unsightly black triangles between the teeth.

Multiple Crowns

Short clinical crowns on multiple teeth may be caused by uncontrolled tooth wear and this is discussed in Chapter 2 and an example shown in Fig 8-6.

Causes of Erosion

It is often difficult to accurately diagnose the causes of erosion. Conversely, it is relatively easy to identify risk factors such as dietary acids. Since acids

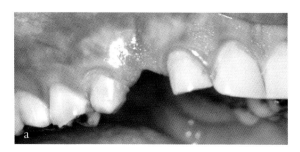

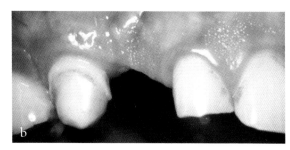

Fig 8-5 (a,b) Surgical crown lengthening apically repositions the gingival margin and increases the length of the clinical crown. Surgery results in the exposure of interdental spaces and may cause black triangles.

are common in the diet, it is often difficult to identify whether the cause of the erosion is the quantity of acid consumed, or more likely, the length of time it is present in the mouth. Holding or swilling a drink in the palatal vault prolongs erosion. Savouring citrus fruits, eating pieces of fruit over an hour or two and placing lemons against the buccal surfaces of upper anterior teeth to provide zest during sports are all known to be associated with an increased risk of erosion. Improving acid clearance by eliminating contributory dietary habits and reducing the frequency of consumption should reduce the risk of further erosion.

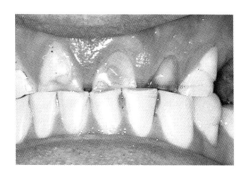

Fig 8-6 Worn anterior teeth caused by erosion and attrition.

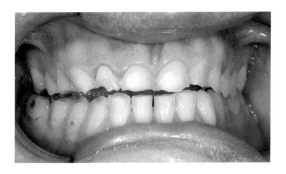

Fig 8-7 The molars on the left side are in contact, but there is an anterior open bite caused by acid erosion. Attrition can not be responsible because of the lack of anterior tooth-to-tooth contact.

Gastric reflux is very common. In affected patients, the acid reflux reaches the mouth, following regurgitation, to cause erosion (Fig 8-7). Typically, tooth wear is severe when this occurs, because the low pH and titratable acidity of the refluxed gastric juice rapidly dissolves the enamel and the dentine. If tooth wear presents in patients who have reflux symptoms which interfere with their quality of life, a referral to a gastroenterologist should be considered. If the tooth wear is severe, but the symptoms of reflux disease are mild, referral to a gastroenterologist is unnecessary.

The role of attrition in tooth wear is often overlooked. If bruxism is identified as the main cause of tooth wear crowns should be prescribed with caution (Fig 8-8 and Fig 8-9). Parafunctional activities cause high occlusal forces; these load small areas of dentine and enamel, producing tooth wear. The high loads placed

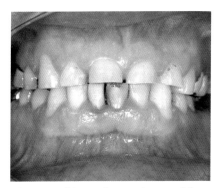

Fig 8-8 This tooth wear is caused by a parafunctional habit of bruxing. The increased loading on the teeth increases the risk of further wear and fracture of restorations.

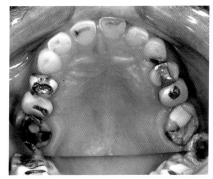

Fig 8-9 The palatal view of the patient seen in Fig 8-8.

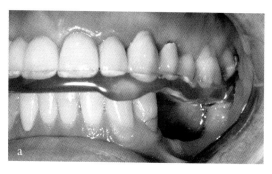

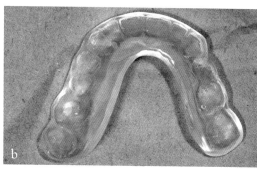

Fig 8-10 (a,b) A full coverage hard acrylic Michigan splint is normally worn at night to protect crowns placed in the management of tooth wear.

on teeth may be damaging to restorations. Under these circumstances, mechanical failure of restorations is more likely, therefore, treating tooth wear caused by attrition can be more risky than that caused by erosion. It is sensible to consider making full coverage hard acrylic splints (Michigan) to protect the teeth and restorations, but the compliance cannot be guaranteed. Careful consideration should be given to whether crowns are the appropriate management. In some situations a pragmatic option is to provide a Michigan splint to prevent further wear and to monitor the tooth wear (Fig 8-10a,b).

Prevention

Most patients do not comply with recommendations to changes in their diet, in particular over the long term. It is therefore sensible to suggest to patients that they subtly alter their diets rather than make drastic changes in the interest of good compliance. Most acidic foods and drinks have the potential to cause dental erosion but those with a high titratable acidity are more likely to be damaging. For example, citrus fruits are particularly erosive whereas common carbonated drinks cause relatively little erosion. The role of fluoride in erosion remains unproven. The fluoride enriched tooth surface has

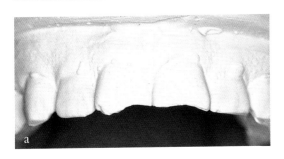

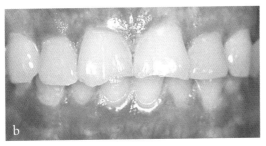

Fig 8-11 (a,b) The two pictures illustrate the slow progression of tooth wear. The study model was obtained 16 years before the clinical photograph. Comparison of the two figures fails to reveal an appreciable progression of wear. In this case monitoring was effective (Courtesy of Prof BGN Smith).

the potential to prevent erosion, but may not be so protective if the eroded surface is immediately removed by abrasion or attrition.

Tooth wear progresses very slowly in most cases, but in some the rate is more rapid. Therefore, for most people a period of monitoring is the most appropriate management, combined with preventive advice. A recent study showed that tooth wear, monitored by study casts progressed very slowly when the patients were given appropriate preventive advice (Bartlett, 2003). In patients in which the rate of wear is relatively fast, restorations may be immediately indicated (Fig 8-11a,b), but it is not currently possible to identify the risk factors which result in rapid tooth wear. Monitoring should start at six-monthly intervals. If no progression is identified the monitoring periods may be extended. The indications when to restore worn teeth are covered in Chapter 2.

Management

Localised Tooth Wear

Localised tooth wear often presents in the upper anterior teeth. The wear produces short teeth without loss of vertical space. Further interocclusal space is needed for crowns or composites and can be created in a number of ways:

- minor axial tooth movement using the Dahl effect

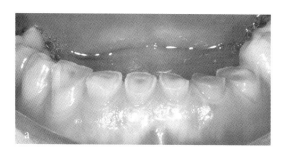

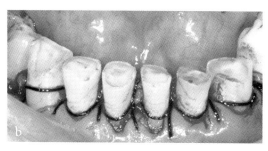

Fig 8-12 (a,b) The cause of the wear on these teeth is bruxism. This has produced short clinical crowns with insufficient crown height for conventional metal-ceramic crowns. Surgical crown lengthening repositioned the gingival margin in an apical direction, increasing the length of the crown.

- crown lengthening
- occlusal adjustment changing the ICP to retruded contact position to create horizontal space between the upper and lower incisors
- conventional orthodontic movement
- reduction of the opposing teeth.

Reduction in the height of the opposing teeth is unwise in patients in which tooth wear has already compromised the dentition. Creating anterior space by repositioning ICP to RCP is possible, but is technically difficult. Diagnostic casts should be mounted in the retruded contact position on a semi-adjustable articulator with the aid of a facebow recording. Adjustments are conducted on the articulated casts until ICP and RCP are coincident. Using the casts as a guide, the same sequence of tooth adjustments is undertaken clinically. This procedure appears simple, but is difficult in practice, and may require a significant amount of occlusal reduction.

Conventional orthodontic treatment can be used to intrude teeth and to create occlusal clearance, but may prove unacceptable to some patients as it is costly and protracted. Crown lengthening increases the length of the clinical crown by apical repositioning of the gingival tissues. The result of crown lengthening on lower incisors is shown in Fig 8-12a and 8-12b. A mucoperiosteal flap is raised, crestal bone removed and the tissue apically repositioned to increase the length of the clinical crown. The surgery exposes interdental spaces and in patients with a high lip line this can prove to be unacceptable.

Minor axial tooth movement by means of splints can create localised interocclusal space, for example in the upper anterior region. Such movement of teeth reverses the effects of dentoalveolar compensation. It has been called the Dahl effect (Fig 8-13a,b). Originally Dahl and co-workers used removable cobalt chrome splints with an anterior bite platform to create space. The technique has been adapted to involve the use of a variety of materials.

Accurate study casts should be mounted on a semiadjustable articulator with the aid of a RCP record. A diagnostic wax-up of the anterior teeth will indicate how much to increase the vertical dimension. The incisal pin is raised to the new vertical dimension and a splint made to restore occlusal contact. Palatally the splint should have a flat bite platform to direct the occlusal forces along the long axis of the teeth (Fig 8-13b). The splint can be cast in metal or made in an indirect composite. It should be cemented to the teeth with a thin mix of glass-ionomer or polycarboxylate luting cement.

The anterior splint separates the posterior teeth. The occlusal forces placed on the splint cause intrusion of the lower anterior teeth, while the posterior

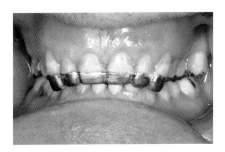

Fig 8-13 (a) A labial view of the Dahl appliance cemented to the anterior teeth. The partial coverage splint contacts the lower anterior teeth but separates the posterior teeth and causes posterior overeruption and intrusion of the anterior teeth. Between 3 to 6 months later the premolars and molars will re-establish an interocclusal contact.

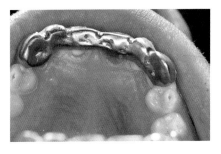

Fig 8-13 (b) The palatal view of the Dahl appliance showing the inter cuspal position contacts.

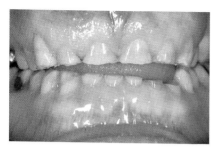

Fig 8-13 (c) With the Dahl appliance removed, sufficient vertical space is available to provide the crowns.

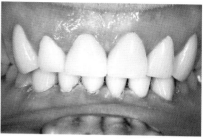

Fig 8-13 (d) The crowns on the upper and lower teeth. The lower anterior teeth are those seen in Fig 8-12.

Fig 8-13 (a-e) The Dahl appliance illustrated allows overeruption of the posterior teeth while causing intrusion of the anterior teeth. Removal of the splint after reversal of alveolar compensation produces sufficient anterior space to accommodate crowns.

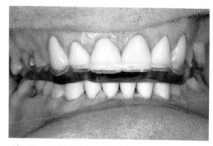

Fig 8-13 (e) Completed crowns are protected from further damage by a Michigan splint.

teeth are allowed to overerupt. After the splint has been in place for a few months the posterior teeth overerupt (60% of the movement) and the anterior teeth are intruded (40% of the movement). At the end of treatment the splint is removed. The interocclusal space created by the splint should be sufficient to restore the worn teeth with crowns without the need for more occlusal reduction. The time taken for the procedure may vary from six to twelve months (Fig 8-13c-e).

Instead of a metal splint, directly placed composites can work in the same way and be more acceptable to the patient (Fig 8-14a,b). Once the vertical space has been created conventional crowns may be used to restore the teeth. Alternatively, composites may be used to form the long-term restorations.

The size of the tooth can be helpful in assessing the success of composite build-ups. Small incisor teeth, such as lower incisors and some upper lateral incisors,

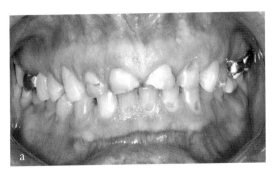

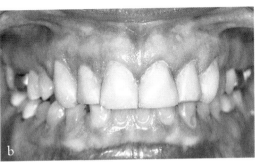

Fig 8-14 (a,b) Directly placed composites can be equally effective as a cast-metal Dahl appliance. These restorations, provided they do not repeatedly fracture, can be used in medium to long-term treatments (By kind permission of Manoj Patel).

have a small surface area which is more susceptible to bond failure (Fig 8-15a,b). This is especially relevant if there is no rim of enamel surrounding the worn tooth, and where the restoration relies completely on the bond to dentine.

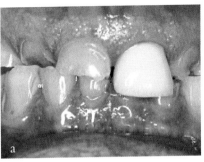

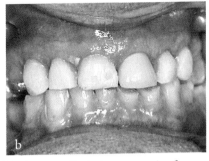

Fig 8-15 (a,b) The presence of small lateral incisors can limit the prognosis of composite build-ups as the surface area is insufficient to retain the composite in the long term. Pretreatment appearance of the worn teeth (a). Appearance of composites used to restore the upper anterior teeth (b). The two lateral incisors suffered repeated fractures and were eventually crowned.

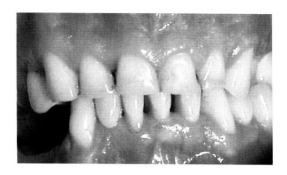

Fig 8-16 Composites have been placed along the incisal edges of the upper anterior teeth. This increased the occlusal vertical dimension and created interocclusal space posteriorly. The space can then be utilised for dentures or implants.

Partially Dentate Patient

If a partially dentate patient has tooth wear, a generalised increase in the occlusal vertical dimension is generally indicated to restore the teeth. In these cases the upper and lower anterior teeth are often retained. This is simpler and quicker than reversing alveolar compensation (Fig 8-16). An absence of posterior teeth is not always associated with more wear occurring on the remaining anterior teeth. Composites may be added to the shortened teeth to restore their shape and increase the vertical dimension. This also produces separation of the posterior edentulous ridges with the possible benefit of increasing the vertical space for dentures. Cold cure acrylic can be added to existing dentures to adapt them to the increased vertical dimension. Composites can be added to teeth in one or both arches. Once an acceptable occlusion and appearance has been achieved with composites, they can be replaced with crowns at a later date.

Generalised Tooth Wear

If the tooth wear is generalised, localised reversal of alveolar compensation is inappropriate and restorations are needed on most contacting teeth (Fig 8-17a-e). It is not necessary for all occluding surfaces to be restored. Often, wear affects some teeth in the upper jaw and some in the lower, and restorations should only normally be placed on those teeth with extensive wear.

Acrylic Splints

Some clinicians recommend an occlusal splint to assess the tolerance of patients to an increased vertical dimension (Fig 8-10b). Such a splint is generally referred to as a Michigan splint and is made on study models mounted on a semiadjustable articulator using a terminal hinge axis occlusal record. This allows the vertical dimension to be increased by raising the incisal pin. The splint should be made in clear heat cured acrylic, with canine risers for lateral excursion. The

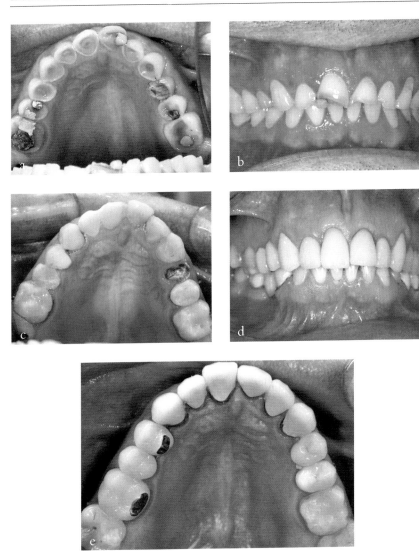

Fig 8-17 (a-e) The tooth wear illustrated has affected all the upper teeth. A full mouth rehabilitation is indicated. Composites can be used to re-establish the vertical dimension, and then employed as cores for conventional crowns.

splint is normally worn in the upper arch. It is important when the splint is fitted that adjustments are made to ensure that all teeth occlude evenly on the splint. This is to ensure that no overeruption of the opposing teeth occurs.

Composite Build-ups

Whilst composites can produce an acceptable result, their long-term success is less assured. Increasingly, directly placed composite restorations are used to assess an increase in the vertical dimension. A diagnostic wax-up is needed to help form and shape the composite restorations. A matrix is made from the wax-up and guides the clinician when adding the composite to the teeth (Fig 8-18a-d).

The width of anterior teeth should be around 80% of tooth length, ensuring that the teeth do not appear too square in shape. An advantage of using a semiadjustable articulator is that the horizontal plane aids in positioning the incisal edges of the teeth.

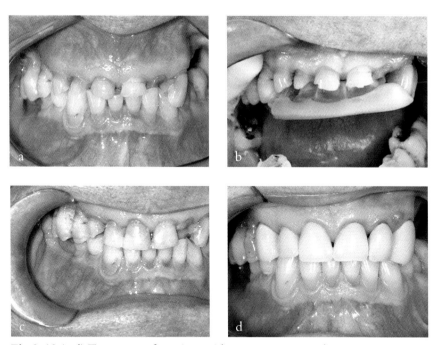

Fig 8-18 (a-d) Treatment of a patient with worn anterior teeth.
Pretreatment appearance of the worn anterior teeth (a). Diagnostic wax-up used to make a silicone matrix to place composite on the worn anterior teeth (b). The vertical dimension increased with directly placed composites (c). Both lateral incisors needed to be root treated and restored with a post-retained crown. Composites established the vertical dimension and tooth shape. After monitoring for a few months the teeth were restored with metal-ceramic crowns (d).

When indicated, composite build-ups can become cores for crowns, provided there is sufficient tooth remaining. The interval between the placement of the composite build-ups and provision of the crowns can vary from months to years. On average, composites used in these situations last around three to five years. The composites are used as diagnostic and transitional restorations. If the patient is satisfied with the lip support, crown height and width, the definitive crowns can be made to reproduce the composites. In some cases the composite restorations may prove to be satisfactory, precluding the need for crowns (Fig 8-14b).

Summary

Management of Tooth Wear
- Determine the aetiology of the tooth wear.
- Start preventive advice and refer to a gastroenterologist as necessary.
- Confirm the patient's main concerns, including:
  - progression of the wear
  - appearance
  - sensitivity.
- Take upper and lower study casts of the patient and examine the teeth for alveolar compensation.
- Mount the casts on a semiadjustable articulator with the aid of a facebow recording. Use the retruded contact position as the interocclusal record.

Localised Tooth Wear
- Make a diagnostic wax-up to create the desired shape and size of the teeth. From the wax-up make a putty matrix.
- The diagnostic wax-up can be copied and a matrix made.
- For localised anterior palatal tooth wear employ the Dahl effect. Use the matrix to help fashion direct composite on the palatal surfaces of the anterior teeth and to control the vertical and horizontal dimensions of the teeth.
- Adjust the provisional restorations to fit the new vertical dimension and ensure that the guidance on the teeth is shared.
- Canine guidance, if applicable, is reproduced.
- After a review period of a few weeks, check the occlusion and adjust if necessary.
- If definitive crowns are planned, the anterior guidance – created by the diagnostic wax-ups can be copied using a custom-formed incisal guidance table on the articulator.
- When using composites as cores ensure that sufficient tooth tissue remains

to act as a ferrule. Insufficient natural tooth may increase the risk of the core material debonding during the provision of crowns. Provided sufficient bulk of tooth remains, this will support the definitive crown.

Generalised Tooth Wear
- Similar to the processes described above.
- Take impressions, facebow recording and occlusal registration in the terminal hinge axis/retruded contact position.
- Make a diagnostic wax-up restoring the short clinical crowns to their original shape and size. Consider a custom-formed incisal guidance table on the articulator.
- Select which teeth are to be restored. This might mean all the teeth in one arch or a combination of teeth in the upper and lower teeth. Normally select the teeth which are most worn.
- From the wax-up either duplicate the model and make a clear vacuum-formed splint or make a putty matrix to aid freehand build-up with composite.
- The wax-up or putty matrix can also be used to make the provisional crowns.
- Prepare the teeth for crowns. This can be undertaken in one or more appointments. For example, anterior teeth can be prepared at the new vertical dimension and provisional crowns fitted. Thereafter, the posterior teeth are prepared and provisional crowns fitted. Finally, an impression is taken of all the preparations and arrangements made to make and fit the crowns together.
- Alternatively, the crowns can be made and fitted in separate stages. Normally, the anterior teeth are restored first to establish the height and shape of the anterior teeth.

Further Reading

Bartlett DW. Retrospective long-term monitoring of tooth wear using study models. Br Dent J 2003;194:211-213.

Ibbetson R, Eder A. Tooth surface loss. London: BDJ books, 2000.

Ricketts DNJ, Smith BGN. Minor axial tooth movement in preparation for fixed prostheses. Eur J Prosthodont Rest Dent 1993;1:145-149.

Ricketts DNJ, Smith BGN. Clinical techniques for producing and monitoring minor axial tooth movement. Eur J Prosthodont Rest Dent 1993;2:5-9.

Chapter 9
When and How to Articulate

Aim

The aim of this chapter is to describe when and how to use an articulator.

Objective

After this chapter the reader will understand when an articulator is necessary in the provision of crowns.

Introduction

Articulating casts is time consuming and costly, but justified in certain cases. It is important to understand what type of articulator to use in these situations. In general, the provision of single restorations and cases in which the casts can be easily located into the ICP, do not need an articulator (Fig 9-1a-c).

There are circumstances when the articulation of casts is important. These include:
- reproducing lateral guidance (Chapter 7)
- occlusal analysis, diagnostic wax-up and trial adjustments
- extensive crowns and bridges with the loss of the intercuspal position.

A frequent question when restoring root-filled canines is: should the occlusion be restored to canine guidance or changed to group function? Converting the guidance to group function can protect the weakened tooth. Removing canine guidance can, however, lead to a short clinical crown with an unacceptable appearance (Fig 9-2). In these situations occlusal adjustment might be required to protect the weakened tooth.

Occlusal Adjustment

Occlusal adjustment can be undertaken before preparation for a crown, or at the time the crown is fitted. Minor occlusal adjustments are often performed at the fit stage; however, the amount required is not always

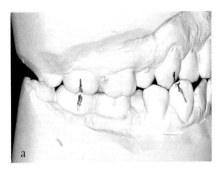
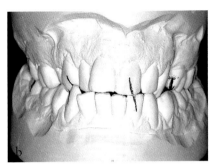
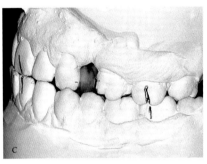

Fig 9-1 (a-c) This patient has an inter-cuspal position which is difficult to record. Pencil marks record where the opposing teeth contact, providing sufficient information to articulate the models. For the construction of most single indirect restorations handheld casts are sufficient.

predictable. In cases in which extensive occlusal adjustment is necessary, this needs to be identified during the preoperative clinical examination. When fitting a crown, unplanned occlusal adjustment of opposing teeth is not good practice, and from a patient standpoint is seen to be an error of judgement. Planned occlusal adjustments should be practised on articulated study models. This allows the amount and nature of the adjustments to be fully appreciated and possibly explained to the patient prior to embarking on the necessary operative procedures. Exposure of dentine,

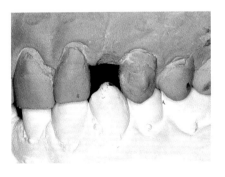

Fig 9-2 This patient has a missing upper canine and the lower canine has overe-rupted. Avoiding heavy occlusal contact in lateral excursions would lead to an unacceptably short pontic. Orthodontic intrusion or adjustment of the lower canine will provide sufficient vertical space to replace the missing tooth. The same applies if the upper canine was compromised by a root filling and post retained core with no ferrule.

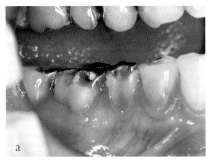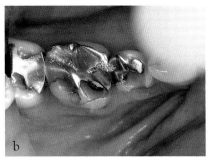

Fig 9-3 (a,b) The worn lower right premolar and molar teeth require replacement gold crowns. The patient has group function in lateral excursions. The use of an articulator will reduce chair-side time required for adjustment of the occlusion.

during adjustments can lead to sensitivity and indicate coronal coverage. In extreme cases elective root canal treatment may be required (Fig 7-3, Chapter 7).

Number of Teeth Being Restored

Restorations placed in patients with group function rather than canine guidance need more clinical time at the fit stage. In these situations, articulated working casts reproduce the movements of the mandible and allow the technician to make all but the final adjustments in the laboratory. This reduces clinical time (Fig 9-3a,b).

The necessity to articulate study and working casts increases with the number of teeth (units) to be crowned. As the number of prepared teeth increases, fewer teeth are available to locate the casts together in the ICP and the risk of errors increases. The choice of articulator type depends upon the clinical situation and complexity of the case. For example, if all the anterior teeth are to be crowned, preserving the anterior guidance, possibly with a custom-formed incisal guidance table requires a semiadjustable articulator (Chapter 7; Fig 7-11).

For crowns on more than one posterior tooth, the choice of articulator depends on the lateral guidance. Handheld, simple hinge or average value articulators are normally sufficient in cases with canine guidance, given disclusion of the posterior teeth in lateral excursion. Whereas, teeth involved in group function tend to require multiple adjustments in the laboratory, justifying the use of a semiadjustable articulator.

Reorganising the Occlusion

When all or most occluding teeth require new restorations, a reorganised approach is indicated. The occlusion is usually reorganised to the terminal hinge axis at a chosen occlusal vertical dimension. A semiadjustable articulator is necessary in such cases (see Chapter 7).

Types of Articulator

There are four main types of articulator, with increasing degrees of complexity.

Simple Hinge

This type of articulator consists of a simple hinge mechanism, linking the upper and lower casts (Fig 9-4). There is no relationship between the anatomical position of the condyles and the occlusal surfaces of the teeth. As a consequence, some adjustment of the cuspal inclines of the restoration may be needed on closure to compensate for the inaccuracy of the articulator. The adjusted crowns will tend to have cusps with reduced height and shallow angles, giving them a relatively flat appearance.

Average Value

The condylar elements on the average value articulator (Fig 9-5) are not anatomically related to the occlusal plane of the teeth. Average value artic-

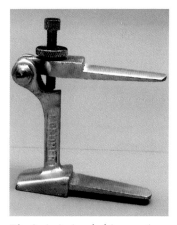

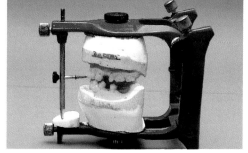

Fig 9-4 A simple hinge articulator.

Fig 9-5 An average value articulator.

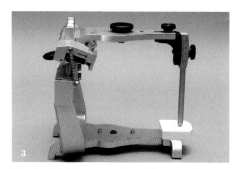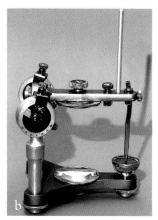

Fig 9-6 (a,b) Semiadjustable articulators. An example of an arcon articulator is illustrated in Fig 9-6a. The articulator shown in Fig 9-6b is a non-arcon articulator.

ulators provide lateral excursive and protrusive movements and have condylar inclinations set to an average value of 30°. The incisive guidance table is usually the only component that can be altered. This type of articulator finds few applications in fixed prosthodontics.

Semiadjustable Articulators

There are two types of semiadjustable articulators, the arcon (Fig 9-6a) and non-arcon (Fig 9-6b).

In the arcon design, the ball or condylar element is attached to the mandibular arm of the articulator and is anatomically correct. Non-arcon articulators have the condylar "ball" attached to the maxillary arm housed in a track connected to the mandibular component. Non-arcon articulators are anatomically incorrect, making it more difficult to appreciate the dynamics of movement of the casts.

A facebow record is normally used to mount the maxillary cast to the upper frame. An ICP or RCP occlusal record is used to mount the mandibular to the maxillary cast. This produces a close approximation of the anatomical relationship between the condyles and the occlusal plane of the teeth. Most semiadjustable articulators allow alteration of the condylar inclination, Bennett angle and movement, and incisal guidance (Fig 9-7).

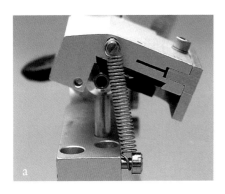
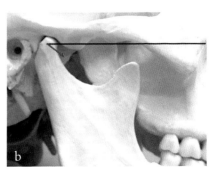
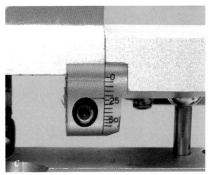
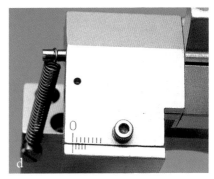
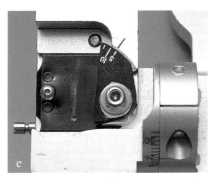

Fig 9-7 (a–e) Adjustable components on the Denar semiadjustable articulator. The lateral view of the condylar element of the articulator and skull shows the condylar guidance (a and b). This can be adjusted by the screw at the back of the articulator to the correct angle on the scale shown (c). Bennett movement (progressive side shift) can be adjusted by the small vernier scale on the top of the condylar element (d), and the Bennett angle (immediate side shift) on the inferior side of the condylar element (e). Intercondylar distance (c) and Fisher angle cannot be set as on the fully adjustable articulator.

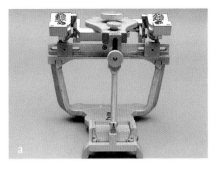
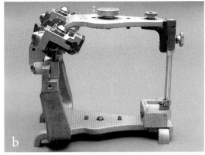
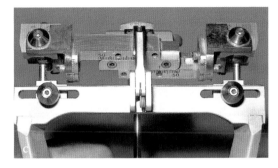

Fig 9-8 (a-c) Anterior (a), lateral (b) and posterior (c) views of a Denar fully adjustable articulator.

Fully Adjustable Articulators (Fig 9-8a-c)

Fully adjustable articulators are very sophisticated devices, but are rarely used. A pantographic facebow records the terminal hinge axis, the position of the condyles and the movement of the condyles. In addition, more adjustments are possible than with a semiadjustable articulator, including changes to the intercondylar width and Fisher angle. Furthermore, condylar inserts can be used to duplicate the curved anatomy of the glenoid fossa. Setting the various values is complicated and technique demanding. As such, fully adjustable articulators are rarely used, even in the most complex of cases.

Facebows

A facebow is a calliper-like device which records the position of the terminal hinge axis relative to the occlusal plane. The facebow recording is used to set the upper cast to the upper arm of the articulator. To do this, three reference points are necessary. The first is the occlusal plane of the upper teeth, the second is the position of the condylar heads when seated in the terminal hinge axis position and the third is the horizontal plane. The horizontal plane is determined from the anterior part of the face. The

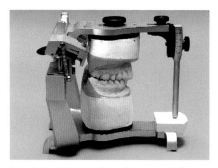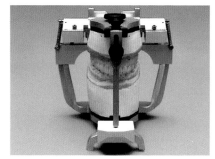

Fig 9-9 Mounted study casts with correct angulation of the occlusal plane.

articulated casts appear as if the patient is sitting or standing upright (Fig 9-9). This helps the technician to make indirect restorations with the correct horizontal plane.

There are a number of facebows on the market which differ slightly in the way reference points are recorded (Fig 9-10 and Fig 9-11). Common to all articulators is a bite fork which is inserted into the mouth. A rigid thermoplastic material records the cusps and incisal edges of the upper teeth. Suitable materials include softened wax, silicone registration pastes or softened impression compound. Only the tips of the teeth need to be recorded. This ensures that the casts will seat fully onto the recording when mounting them to the upper arm of the articulator. The bite fork is usually positioned to the right of the patient's mid-line to allow space for the incisal pin of the articulator during mounting of the casts.

To record the true terminal hinge axis position, a hinge axis locator or kinematic facebow is needed. This consists of clutches, held rigidly to the maxillary

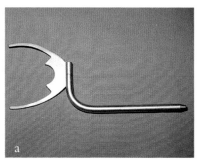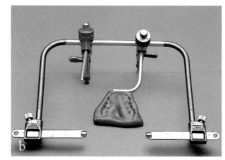

Fig 9-10 Dentatus bitefork (a) and assembled facebow with orbital pointer (b).

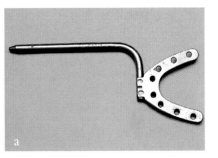

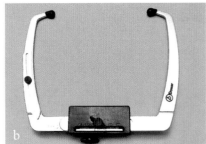

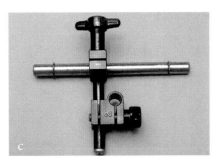

Fig 9-11 (a-c) Denar Slidematic earbow with bite fork (notch anteriorly to align with the central incisor contact point) (a), earbow (b) and jig (c).

and mandibular teeth. The lower clutch is attached to a facebow with adjustable side arms. The length and angulation of the arms can be adjusted as the patient opens and closes in the terminal hinge axis position. This is done until the hinge axis pointers rotate only, with no arcing (Fig 9-12). The true terminal hinge axis can then be marked on the skin with a pen or skin pencil.

The true terminal hinge axis position must be identified when using a fully adjustable articulator. Such articulators are rarely used in practice.

A number of arbitrary hinge axis positions have been described. A position 13 mm from posterior margin of the tragus to a line on the outer canthus of the eye is probably the most commonly used and reasonably accurate. The bitefork and impression material are pressed firmly against the occlusal surfaces of the maxillary teeth and loosely attached to the facebow. The condylar rods of the facebow are adjusted until they rest on the skin over the skin marks. The facebow has a millimetre scale marked onto the condylar rods. The bow is moved along these rulers from side to side, until the same reading is obtained on both sides. The screws are then tightened (Fig 9-13a-d). This ensures that the head is centrally placed within the facebow. With the bitefork locked securely in place, the third reference point can be recorded.

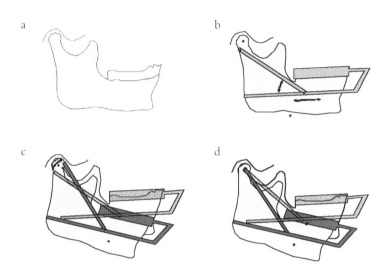

Fig 9-12 Diagrammatic representation of how a kinematic facebow is used. An impression of the lower dental arch is taken in a tray which is attached to a facebow (a,b). The arms of the bow can be extended, and the angulation altered until the condylar pointer no longer arches (c) on opening and closing in the terminal hinge axis position (d).

For the Dentatus articulator and facebow, an orbital pointer, loosely attached to the bow, is moved to touch the skin over the infraorbital notch and locked into place. This information fixed within the facebow can then be transferred to the articulator.

Recording the arbitrary hinge axis position and centralising the facebow is time consuming and can lead to errors. Slidematic earbows have been designed to overcome such problems. An example is the Denar facebow (Waterpik Technologies, USA). As the bow is closed the plastic ear pieces are placed into the external auditory meatuses, centralising the patient's head within the bow and allowing the intercondylar distance to be recorded (Fig 9-11 and Fig 9-14a-f). With the bitefork positioned on the maxillary teeth, and loosely attached to the correctly positioned bow via the mounting jig, the third reference point can be recorded. This point lies on the skin to the side of the nose, 43 mm above the incisal edge of the lateral incisor teeth. The facebow is rotated up or down until the reference pointer is aligned with the mark. The jig is tightened and the slidematic facebow is opened and removed from the patient. The jig and bitefork are required by the laboratory to articulate the upper cast.

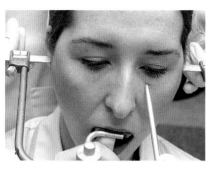
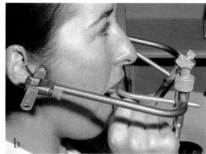
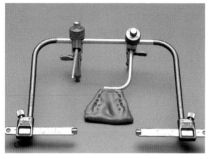
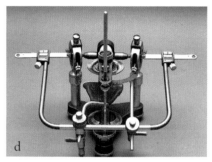

Fig 9-13 (a-d) Mounting the maxillary cast on a Dentatus articulator. The bitefork is covered in wax and an imprint of the teeth recorded. The facebow is attached and the condylar pointers placed over the marked arbitrary hinge axis position (a,b). The facebow is centralised by sliding the facebow side to side until the rulers give the same left and right readings. The bow is tightened and the third reference point (most inferior part of the orbital rim, the orbitale) recorded using the orbital pointer. The bite fork and orbital pointer screws are tightened and the condylar pointers are released for removal (c). The facebow is transferred to the articulator and the condylar pointers placed over the condylar heads and the bow moved until both rulers give the same reading. The bow is lowered or raised until the orbital pointer is level with the articulator's orbital plane (d). The upper cast can now be seated onto the bite-fork and mounted into place with anti-expansion plaster.

Interocclusal Records

Terminal Hinge Axis Record

The mandibular cast is mounted on the articulator, and its relationship with the maxillary cast dictated by the interocclusal record. This record should be taken to avoid any tooth contacts and the risk of sliding into ICP rather than the terminal hinge position. The mandible is guided into the terminal hinge axis position by asking the patient to open and close to produce pure rotation movement around the hinge axis. In some patients, it is difficult to

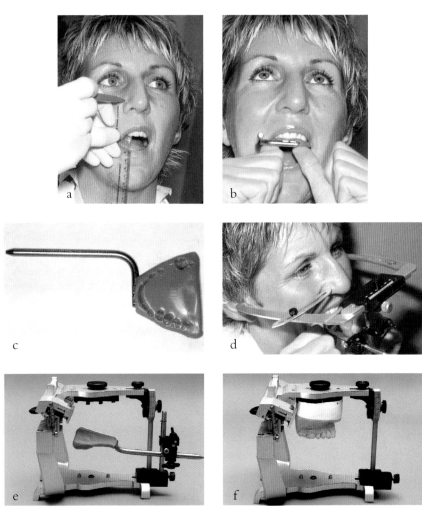

Fig 9-14 (a–f) Mounting the maxillary cast on a Denar semiadjustable articulator. First, the third reference point (43 mm from the incisal edge of the upper lateral incisor) is marked on the side of the nose (a). The bitefork is covered in softened wax and an imprint of the tips of the upper teeth recorded (b,c). This is held in situ by the patient whilst the jig and earbow are assembled (d) and the height of the bow adjusted until the reference pointer is level with the marked position on the nose. Once the screws numbered 1 and 2 are tightened the earbow can be released. The jig and bitefork are then removed from the earbow and are securely placed into a mounting plate on the articulator (e). The upper cast can then be seated into the wax imprint and set into position on a mounting plate using anti-expansion plaster (f).

guide the mandible into this position given muscle tension or learnt paths of closure. In such circumstances occlusal splints or incisal jigs can be used to break the conditioned path of closure. Taking a terminal hinge axis record becomes all the more important with increases in the number of indirect units being made, and when a reorganised approach is adopted for a full arch rehabilitation.

Intercuspal Record

Single unit restorations, which conform to the existing occlusion, do not necessitate the use of complex articulators, if any, and can often be made by hand holding the models. When providing restorations in some complex cases, a semiadjustable articulator is required and additional occlusal records may need to be taken to set the condylar inclination, Bennett angle and Bennett shift.

Setting the Condylar Inclination

As a patient moves into protrusion, the condyles move forwards and downwards onto the articular eminence, resulting in disclusion of the posterior teeth. The relationship of the anterior teeth dictates the stage at which, and to what extent, the posterior teeth disclude. At the extremes, anterior teeth in a Class III incisor relationship contribute little, if any, or no posterior disclusion. Conversely, anterior teeth in a Class II Division II contribute considerably to the disclusion of the posterior teeth. The movement of the mandible in protrusion is governed by posterior–skeletal and anterior–tooth determinants. Obtaining a protrusive interocclusal record to record the degree of posterior tooth disclusion and moving the articulated casts until they seat perfectly into this record allows the left and right condylar inclination to be set.

Bennett Settings

In lateral excursions, the mandible moves towards the working side. The initial element of this movement is the immediate side shift and is measured at the working condyle. The non-working condyle, as viewed from above, moves forwards and medially in an arc of curvature centred around the working condyle. When viewed in this plane the angle with the sagittal plane is called the Bennett angle (Fig 7-6b, Chapter 7). To measure this, left and right lateral excursive interocclusal records are needed.

Rather than taking a series of interocclusal records to set the condylar inclination, Bennett angle and Bennett shift, some manufacturers have introduced electronic devices similar to a facebow to determine these values.

149

Interocclusal Records

Impressions of the teeth should be as accurate as possible. Air blows in the occlusal surfaces, typically in fissures, will result in beads on the die stone and prevent accurate seating of the interocclusal record. There is no need to use an interocclusal record if the working casts can be easily located in the ICP. To help with the location, pencil marks on the cast allow the technician to see where the teeth interdigitate (Fig 9-1).

Occlusal records are needed when articulating to the terminal hinge axis position, or when the ICP is unclear. The two most commonly used interocclusal materials are waxes and polyvinyl siloxanes. When softened wax is used, this should not be rolled into a horseshoe shape to cover the occlusal surfaces, as cross arch distortion can occur. If this happens, it is not possible to return the wax to its original shape. A double thickness of a hard wax is preferred which, when cooled, is more rigid. The wax should also cross the

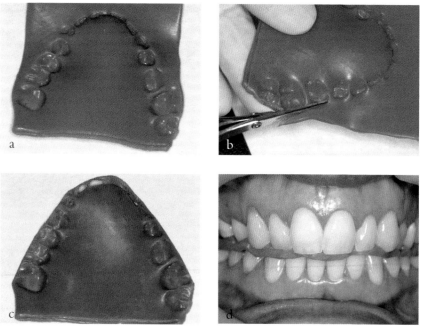

Fig 9-15 (a–d) The stages involved in making a wax interocclusal record. A double layer of wax is used (a), trimmed along the line of the buccal cusps (b,c) and reseated to correct any distortion as a result of the trimming procedure (d).

arch (Fig 9-15a-d). The record can be reinforced by incorporating a wire mesh. Once the occlusion has been recorded, the wax should be trimmed to the buccal cusps. This allows the technician to ensure complete seating of the casts in the laboratory. Trimming will distort the wax and, as a consequence, the interocclusal record should be resoftened and reseated. For greater accuracy, the upper and lower surfaces of the occlusal record can be smeared with a zinc oxide and eugenol temporary cement and reseated intra-orally until set. Thereafter the record should be disinfected, kept cool and positioned on the casts to avoid distortion.

A disadvantage of using wax is the potential for irreversible distortion and inaccurate occlusal registration if the wax is insufficiently softened. This disadvantage is overcome by silicone registration materials which are injected over the occlusal surfaces. The rapid set of the silicone reduces the possibility of error caused by patient and operator fatigue when recording a pre-contact terminal hinge axis position (Fig 9-16a-c).

Soft registration materials can distort on seating the opposing casts whereas harder registration materials are easier to use and allow a more accurate registration. In some situations where indirect restorations are being made for patients with extensive edentulous areas, occlusal rims are required to articulate the casts.

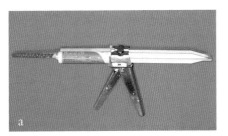
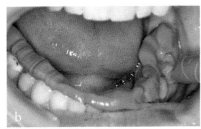

Fig 9-16 (a-c) A silicone occlusal registration paste with a double helix mixer tip to produce an even mix with no air inclusions (a). The flattened mixer tip ensures a wide deposit of material onto the occlusal surfaces (b) into which the patient closes (c).

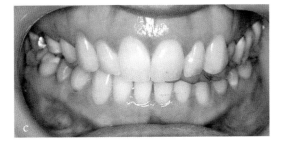

Checking the Occlusion

When trying-in indirect restorations, it is important to check the marginal fit and contact areas. These are critical, as poor fit or a tight contact compromises the restoration. The seating of the restoration needs to be checked and adjusted prior to examining the occlusion. Both can be checked with pressure relief sprays such as Occlude (Pascal, USA) (Fig 9-17), which is rubbed off tight contacts when the restoration is placed and removed. Following successful adjustment and seating, the occlusion should be checked in ICP and all excursive movements. The occlusal stops on adjacent teeth, and on the contralateral side, should also be checked with and without the crown to confirm that they conform to the ICP. Placing multiple units requires greater care and time. This should be accomplished by adjusting the crowns, one at a time, to the ICP. If necessary try-in individual crowns with and without the adjacent restorations in place. Adjust the crowns until all the units conform to the planned occlusal relationship.

In contrast to gross errors which result in separation of the teeth, small errors are difficult to detect without using articulator paper. Firstly, the patient's perception of a "high" restoration should be checked. Some patients with anaesthetised teeth find this task difficult. A telltale sign of a "high" restoration is the sound when the patient is asked to tap the teeth together. If the restoration interferes with the occlusion in ICP a dull sound can be heard. This is in contrast to the high pitched clash of teeth when the restoration is not in place. Placing a finger on the buccal aspect of the crown when the patient taps their teeth together can also give valuable information. A high restoration can be detected by fremitus or slight mobility on contact.

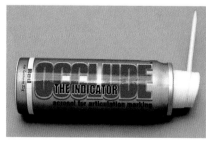

Fig 9-17 Occlude spray used to assess the quality of contact areas and the fit surface of indirect restorations.

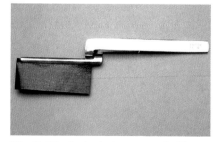

Fig 9-18 Articulating paper held in a Miller holder.

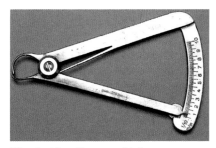

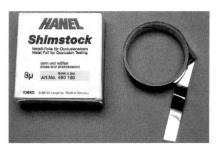

Fig 9-19 Crown thickness gauge. Always check that the gauge reads zero before use, i.e. the gauge illustrated has been distorted.

Fig 9-20 Shimstock foil for checking the occlusion.

Clinical assessments, whilst useful, are crude and subjective and, as such, should be carried out in conjunction with the use of articulating paper. Thin articulating papers are much more sensitive and helpful than thicker varieties, which may result in excessive adjustment. Articulating papers can conveniently be held in a Miller holder, thereby ensuring that the paper is flat and extends to the posterior part of the mouth without folding over (Fig 9-18). It is important that the teeth and restorations are dry, otherwise pressure points will not be marked. A high restoration should be adjusted in the ICP until even occlusal contacts occur on both the restoration being checked and the adjacent teeth. When adjustments to an occlusal surface are indicated, the thickness of the crown should be checked continually throughout adjustment with a crown thickness gauge (Fig 9-19). This ensures that the crown does not become too thin (<0.3 mm) with the risk of perforation. If there is a risk of perforation, consider remaking the restoration, or possibly making adjustments to the opposing teeth.

Excessive occlusal adjustment which leaves a restoration out of occlusion should be avoided. This can lead to a non-functional restoration and an unstable occlusion. To ensure that the restoration is in functional occlusion and not "high", it is advisable to use Shimstock foil (Roeko, Germany) as illustrated in Fig 9-20 and Fig 9-21.

Once contacts in ICP have been adjusted, excursive contacts should be examined. Excursive contacts can be differentiated from ICP contacts by using articulating papers of different colours. Restorations in group function or anterior guidance should be checked for even occlusal contact with the adjacent teeth. In lateral excursions, the non-working side should be

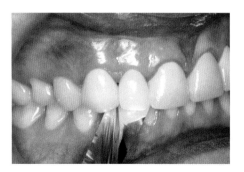

Fig 9-21 Shimstock foil being used to check the occlusion on upper anterior crowns. In intercuspal position the crowns are in contact as the foil cannot be removed. However, the crowns could be "high" and therefore the foil should be moved to between the premolar teeth, when again, there should be firm contact and the foil should not be able to be pulled from between the teeth.

checked to ensure no adverse non-working side interferences have been introduced.

Following all necessary adjustments, the restoration should be polished. This is particularly important if ceramic has been adjusted, as rough, unglazed ceramic surfaces can cause considerable wear of the opposing teeth.

Further Reading

Klineberg I, Jagger R. Occlusion and Clinical Practice: an Evidence-based approach. London: Wright, 2004.

Index

Quintessentials for General Dental Practitioners Series

in 50 volumes

Editor-in-Chief: Professor Nairn H F Wilson

The Quintessentials for General Dental Practitioners Series covers basic principles and key issues in all aspects of modern dental medicine. Each book can be read as a stand-alone volume or in conjunction with other books in the series.

Publication date, approximately

Clinical Practice, Editor: Nairn Wilson

Culturally Sensitive Oral Healthcare	available
Dental Erosion	available
Special Care Dentistry	available
Evidence Based Dentistry	Spring 2007
Dental Bleaching	Spring 2007
Infection Control for the Dental Team	Spring 2007
Therapeutics and Medical Emergencies in the Everyday Clinical Practice of Dentistry	Summer 2007

Oral Surgery and Oral Medicine, Editor: John G Meechan

Practical Dental Local Anaesthesia	available
Practical Oral Medicine	available
Practical Conscious Sedation	available
Minor Oral Surgery in Dental Practice	available

Imaging, Editor: Keith Horner

Interpreting Dental Radiographs	available
Panoramic Radiology	available
Twenty-first Century Dental Imaging	Summer 2007

Periodontology, Editor: Iain L C Chapple

Understanding Periodontal Diseases: Assessment and Diagnostic Procedures in Practice	available
Decision-Making for the Periodontal Team	available
Successful Periodontal Therapy – A Non-Surgical Approach	available
Periodontal Management of Children, Adolescents and Young Adults	available
Periodontal Medicine: A Window on the Body	available

Endodontics, Editor: John M Whitworth

Rational Root Canal Treatment in Practice	available
Managing Endodontic Failure in Practice	available
Restoring Endodontically Treated Teeth	Spring 2007

Prosthodontics, Editor: P Finbarr Allen

Teeth for Life for Older Adults	available
Complete Dentures – from Planning to Problem Solving	available
Removable Partial Dentures	available
Fixed Prosthodontics in Dental Practice	available
Occlusion: A Theoretical and Team Approach	Spring 2007
Managing Orofacial Pain in Practice	Summer 2007

Operative Dentistry, Editor: Paul A Brunton

Decision-Making in Operative Dentistry	available
Aesthetic Dentistry	available
Communicating in Dental Practice	available
Indirect Restorations	available
Choosing and Using Dental Materials	Spring 2007
Composite Restorations in Posterior Teeth	Summer 2007

Paediatric Dentistry/Orthodontics, Editor: Marie Therese Hosey

Child Taming: How to Manage Children in Dental Practice	available
Paediatric Cariology	available
Treatment Planning for the Developing Dentition	available
Managing Dental Trauma in Practice	available

General Dentistry and Practice Management, Editor: Raj Rattan

The Business of Dentistry	available
Risk Management in General Dental Practice	available
Quality Matters: From Clinical Care to Customer Service	available
Practice Management for the Dental Team	Summer 2007

Dental Team, Editor: Mabel Slater

Team Players in Dentistry	Summer 2007

Implantology, Editor: Lloyd J Searson

Implantology in General Dental Practice	available

Quintessence Publishing Co. Ltd., London